BEYOND
NINE
MONTHS

Get Renewed Confidence in Your Body So You Can Feel Like Yourself Again...Months or Years after Childbirth!

Best Ways to Solve
Prolapse - Bladder Leakage- Back Pain
Abdominal Separation - Painful Sex

Dr. Dawn D. Andalon, PT, DPT, MTC, CPI

Publisher: *LEVEL4 Physical Therapy & Performance, Inc.,*

171 Saxony Rd. Ste.105, Encinitas, CA 92024.

While they have made every effort to verify the information here, neither the author nor the publisher assumes any responsibility for errors in, omissions from or a different interpretation of the subject matter. This information may be subject to varying laws and practices in different areas, states, and countries. The reader assumes all responsibility for the use of the information.

Every effort has been made to make this book as accurate as possible. Any errors or inconsistencies are unintentional. The purpose of this book is to inform and educate. No individual should use the information in this book for self-diagnosis, treatment or as justification for accepting or declining any medical therapy for any health problem or disease. No individual is discouraged from seeking professional medical advice and treatment. This book is not supplying medical advice. Any implication of the information herein is at the reader's own risk. Any individual with a specific health problem should first seek advice from his or her personal physician or healthcare provider before starting any program of self-care, especially one that includes a change in diet or level of exercise. The author and publisher shall in no event be held liable to a party for any damages arising directly or indirectly from any use of this material.

ISBN - 9781688328815

Edited by: Amy J. Haywood
Cover photography by: Petula Pea Photography

TESTIMONIALS

Beyond Nine Months is the perfect resource for women looking for answers on how best to heal from having a baby. Whether it has been weeks, months, or years since your delivery, there are things you can do to optimize your recovery. Dr. Dawn Andalon lays out the path to recovery in a concise, easy to follow way. She is passionate about making sure women achieve the healthy, active life they deserve without fear of symptoms and issues. Beyond Nine Months is a must read for all women who either plan to enter or are already part of this race we call motherhood.

— Brooke Kalisiak PT, DPT WCS, Owner of Legacy Physical Therapy

Dr. Andalon highlights something in motherhood that is so important, that once you become a mother you are always postpartum. Women have been taught by society to not talk about how our bodies really change once we have babies, and, therefore, important issues we face in regards to our wellness are overlooked. But, Dr. Andalon believes and teaches women it is never too late to start taking care of you, no matter how many years postpartum you may be! This is a must read for any postpartum mama looking to put her wellness first, so she can, in turn, give back to those she loves most and live her life with confidence!"

— Lara Schulte, Co-Founder, Generation.Mom

After my pregnancy, I had a pretty severe umbilical hernia and a diastasis. I consulted with a surgeon and quickly had the hernia repaired at five months postpartum. I REALLY wish I had waited and consulted with a pelvic floor PT before I rushed to the surgery option. Because the surgeon did a poor job, I've been told that I'm not a candidate for any sort of plastic surgery to fix the skin, and the doctor did not give me instruction on scar mobility. Dr. Dawn helped me eight years later with exercises to help my diastasis. I was amazed after one session how much tighter my ab area felt.

— Amy, 42 (former client)

If you are a new momma or pregnant, or even years into the postpartum journey, Dawn is an excellent resource for all levels and can help you reach your goals. Whether you are a competitive athlete or just learning how to move well and feel more confident with your body, Dawn knows her stuff! She helped me work through my incontinence, pelvic floor heaviness and navigated the process for learning how to work on strengthening my pelvic floor and breathing techniques. Before working with Dr. Dawn, it was a definite that when I would perform certain movements, I would leak or feel heaviness, and now I am able to use the strategies I learned and continue to build my pelvic floor strength to be able to do those movements, symptom free! I am so happy that I worked with her and will be reaching out to her again for my pregnancy work out guidance!

— Korina, 28 (former client)

I started seeing Dr. Dawn about 4 months after the birth of my 2nd son. My first son was 11 lbs and my 2nd was 9 lbs. Both were delivered via C-section and they both did a number on my abdomen. I was having daily lower back pain and knew my diastasis recti (DR) needed to be rehabbed properly before I jumped back into exercise. I had tried pretty much every online program/DVD/wrap/etc. you can think of and had seen another PT after my first son. After a couple of sessions with Dawn, I quickly realized that I had been doing core exercises incorrectly/ineffectively. It's been a couple months since I started and my core is SO much stronger. She also helped me understand that I'm able to do so much more than I thought with my DR as long as I'm conscious of my form and breathing. I have a strong foundation of knowledge from which to build and the confidence to keep going thanks to Dr. Dawn. It's the absolute best gift you can give yourself postpartum!

— Jodi, 35 (former client)

CONTENTS

ACKNOWLEDGEMENTS

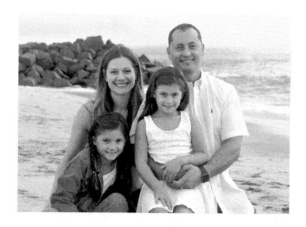

I can't go without thanking my husband and business partner, Oscar, who no matter what sees my potential and pushes me to reach the best version of myself daily.

Also, to our two sweet girls (Alexa & Sophia) who asked me weekly if my book was done yet.
I hope I can be the best female role model for you girls and make you proud!

To my editor and one of my best friends, Amy, who met me just weeks after we became moms for the first time. You inspired me with your questions and helped me find my purpose as a physical therapist to specialize in women's health.

And finally, our business consultant and overall amazing role model, Paul Gough (and his team!), for keeping us set on our goals and coaching us along the way!

INTRODUCTION

What Moms Wish They Knew (But Are Rarely Told)

I wrote this book for you; the mom you want to be and the mom you are meant to be! In this book, I will bring you awareness and clarity, plus give you the confidence you need to maximize your female physical health, especially after childbirth (no matter what your age!).

*Our society tends to praise and admire women who bounce back so quickly after having a baby, who got their "body back," and who simply jumped back into their old fitness routine. That's the pressure we have on ourselves, the pressure we feel instead of praising our bodies for what they have accomplished. The amount of tangible information out there for moms is minimal (especially in the first steps of recovery after childbirth). We should be restoring our bodies to be able to perform as a **stronger and even more confident version of ourselves** and be given a more tactical guide to follow. My hope is this book serves as that missing link for you, no matter what stage you are in life as a mother.*

Usually the motivation to write a book on a topic means the author has a vast amount of knowledge on or has a driving personal experience that led her/him to even consider writing a book...let's just say I have both.

In more than 15 years of practicing as a physical therapist (PT), I have encountered thousands of women of all different ages and backgrounds, which has helped motivate my vision of getting this information out into the public, I am a mom of two who saw firsthand the gap between labor/delivery and postpartum support and educational material on what to expect in your body after you have a baby. Being a physical therapist, you would think I had more in my brain to help with this, but I struggled even to help myself and was often surprised I had to really seek out and research what to do next...and it was my own body!

After two vaginal deliveries, both very different, I struggled with a significant abdominal separation after I delivered my second child who was 9 pounds, 2 ounces; and I had excruciating pelvic pain when walking and climbing stairs that took a few months to resolve. The typical situation is: You see your OB/GYN approximately six weeks postpartum, and if you are medically "healed," you are told you are in the clear, and it's okay to go back to exercise.

My question after that six-week check-in was: "When was I going to feel like myself again?" But I was healed, right?! My friends having babies were asking me questions about problems they were experiencing, and these same issues were being discussed in mom groups I attended. One huge commonality I kept seeing among women was that they were dismissing their issues and accepting them as "side effects" of having a baby.

My interest in women's health started early in my career, but a new direction within physical therapy began after the birth of our first daughter. What I had thought was pressure from society and its hurry-up-and-get-back-into-shape mentality, was really part of the lack of support and guidance for moms when it comes to recovery and physical health in the fourth trimester. With my being a PT and fitness enthusiast, you would think I'd have had more in my toolbox. We were lectured for a whole two hours in graduate school on the pelvic floor and women's health PT; but, really, how would I have known?

"If you check the health of a woman, you check the health of society."

– Rebecca Milner

In a national survey, about one third of mothers who received a postpartum checkup felt their health concerns were not addressed[1]. Common physical pelvic and abdominal problems that most new mothers encountered over the first six months were not identified or addressed in the regular postpartum checkup.

A staggering 91 percent of women post-pregnancy experience some sort of birth-related symptoms that are NOT completely gone by six weeks postpartum. 91 percent!! That just blows my mind, but I believe it based on what I have seen in my office. I would have chosen a different direction in my career path if I had not experienced this firsthand, myself, as a woman. The journey to this place where I am educating and speaking about these topics comes from years of hearing stories straight from the clients I have had the pleasure of helping and the endless phone calls and events where I have been approached by women sharing their stories.

Increased prevalence of postnatal pain and physical issues have been noted in women in the immediate postpartum periods and at several years postpartum. In addition to fatigue, tiredness, and pain, other physical conditions of lower prevalence have a significant impact on mothers' physical and social health. Such conditions include hemorrhoids,

---

[1] Declercq E. R. et al. *Listening to mothers: Report of the first national U.S. survey of women's childbearing experiences.* New York: Maternity Center Association, 2002.

constipation, urinary incontinence, disturbed sleep, lack of sexual desire, and painful intercourse, just to name a few.[2]

The medical system feeds women volumes of information about pre- and post- pregnancy, pre- and post- menopausal symptoms, urinary incontinence, pelvic floor pain, pelvic floor prolapse, diastasis recti, painful intercourse, low back pain, leaking during exercise, and many other subjects, but the system provides almost no information about what women can do about these issues. This is simultaneously frightening and disempowering. It is like telling women they have a ticking time bomb inside. Whether you are a female dealing with breast or ovarian cancer, for instance, most current medical providers will ask you to come back once a year so they can see if it's gone off, but they will rarely tell you how you can defuse it.

This book is a guide to help pregnant and postpartum women of ALL ages and backgrounds. Postpartum recovery is neglected in the United States and is quite different from care in other parts of the world; it leaves women with less time and care to focus solely on postpartum healing. I want to reach the mom (of all ages!) who values her health, no matter what, and realizes she must take care of herself so she can be the best version of the woman she was meant to be; in turn, this will free her to be a much better mom and wife.

Women often see me in their 40s and beyond after the focus is no longer on their babies and toddlers and they're finding more time to prioritize their health now that the kids are in school. Regardless of age, though, it's important to know that when it comes to recovery, IT IS NEVER TOO

---

[2] Thompson, Jane F., et al. "Prevalence and Persistence of Health Problems After Childbirth: Associations with Parity and Method of Birth." Birth, vol. 29, no. 2, 16 May 2002, pp. 83–94., doi:10.1046/j.1523-536x.2002.00167.x.

LATE! Even though I reference the "postpartum" mom, really, it could be months and even YEARS since you had your kids, and now you're wanting to become the best possible version of yourself, which includes attending to your physical FEMALE health.

To be frank, the healthcare availability and advice given to postpartum women in this country following delivery of babies sickens me. Women in the United States oftentimes are left guessing what is next, wishing they knew what to expect with postpartum recovery; and if any symptom arises, they are searching online for answers. Countries such as France, for example, focus a lot more nurturing and standard care in the postpartum period with longer maternity leave, pelvic floor rehabilitation in follow up weeks, and planned restorative exercise classes. One positive change in the U.S. happened in May 2018 when the American College of Obstetricians and Gynecologists updated its guidelines to support improved maternal care and encourage postpartum contact with the medical provider within three weeks postpartum, rather than the typical six to eight weeks. I have yet to see that fully change; the gap in time after labor and delivery and a check-in with a medical provider still leaves women with a lot of time trying to figure things out on their own.[3]

Many women are vulnerable to further medical complications and frustrated because they feel lost in their own bodies; it might even have affected their relationships, and they are living with unanswered questions. Pelvic floor physical therapy is an option that many women don't even know exists unless their OB/GYN or midwife knows to refer to one (and not many do). This is why I have dedicated this book to women as a guide to

---

[3] Cheng, Ching-Yu, et al. "Postpartum Maternal Health Care in the United States: A Critical Review." *Journal of Perinatal Education*, vol. 15, no. 3, 2006, pp. 34–42., doi:10.1624/105812406x119002.

help answer some of the common questions I get asked as a women's health and pelvic floor specialist.

Mental/emotional and physical health and wellbeing are the pillars of thriving in motherhood. For my clients, I emphasize all of these, but for the purpose of this book we will focus mainly on just one of these pillars because, as a PT, it is my specialty. When you look at our current system and resources provided to new moms, they emphasize care for the new baby, breastfeeding, how to manage your life as a mom, support for postpartum depression (although this still needs a lot more awareness and support), and sleep. These are all common topics offered in classes or through outside support.

But really, let's talk about the physical health of the MOM for once. We train for races and competitions—but for motherhood?? We train to get our bodies to look or perform a certain way, but do we train to restore, heal, and perform for the demands of motherhood following a nine-month period that has put a significant strain on our physical body?

Exercise for the new mom often seems difficult because she is too darn exhausted OR she has a very cute infant attached to her 24-7. Then, when kids are older and exercise and self-care become more of a priority, many times I've seen women go back to their old routines. Lack of proper training becomes an issue when now they are facing symptoms of pelvic heaviness, back pain, leaking when they run or jump, and other symptoms they didn't notice as much before!

So, after a six-week postpartum checkup most OB/GYNs will advise, "Ok, you are good to go, clear to exercise again!" This was my experience (and my own OB knew I was a PT) and that of thousands of other women with whom I have spoken. We all felt like there was a missing piece. What if, *instead, doctors said, "Ok, next step is to make an appointment to talk to a pelvic floor PT to get your physical self restored and stronger so you CAN go back to doing exercise properly"?*

Checking for pelvic floor muscle strength; assessing for pelvic organ prolapse and function to help control bowel and bladder control; teaching proper care for a C-section scar to prevent adhesions to the muscle system beneath; building a solid "core" foundation to prevent postnatal back pain; and checking for a diastasis recti (abdominal separation) or abdominal hernia are assessment pieces that are integral to a woman's recovery and prevention of long-term issues. In the United States today, these are NOT typical parts of an OB/GYN's postpartum assessment.

POSTPARTUM HEALTHCARE IN COUNTRIES OUTSIDE THE UNITED STATES

I did a little research on what happens in other countries, and it's pretty mind-blowing. How women are cared for in other cultures and societies, what extra support they are given, and the importance placed on postnatal physical recovery is prioritized. Healthcare professionals in all northern and western European countries provide home visits after childbirth. For example, in the Netherlands, women with normal pregnancies can give birth at home or in birth rooms, which are operated by midwives or general practitioners in a hospital. A continuous one-week home care program covered by insurance for normal birth mothers is provided by a specialist, who receives a three-year training program. This postpartum home care includes care for children and mothers—and housework services.

Despite home visits, mothers can also choose to stay in maternity centers for postpartum care. In Norway, maternity centers established near hospitals are hotel-like environments where new mothers, newborns, and their families can stay together for postpartum care. Likewise, in Taiwan, new mothers can choose to stay in private maternity centers where mothers and newborns are taken care of by nurses. A majority of Chinese mothers who choose to stay at home are cared for by their family members for about one month to prevent diseases and promote health.

*Parental leave is another policy that facilitates maternal and child health. In Sweden, new parents can take, at most, a one-year leave while retaining 80 percent of their salary.[4] Incredible! Even 20 years ago in Finland, mothers had the chance to take a one-year maternal leave supported by a state grant.[5] Whether provided at home or in a facility, postpartum care helps new mothers to **recover from physical changes of pregnancy** and to learn childcare skills.*

Mostly in the USA we have a reactive system rather than proactive system; doctors have less and less time with their patients, unable to really "listen" and offer alternative options outside of a magic "pill," a surgery, an injection, or, worst of all, telling the patient to "wait and see if it gets better on its own." In their defense, their goal is to find red flags, keep their patients medically stable, and help prevent and cure diseases. For some medical providers, it might be that they lack understanding of other resources that could actually provide a significant amount of good to their patients. Other times, in the technology era we exist in, "Dr. Google" may be a quicker resource for women who may not be inclined to see their doctor for a specific concern and instead do their own research on what is happening to their body. Additionally, a gap in care exists between the six-

[4] Vries, Raymond De, et al. *Birth by Design: Pregnancy, Maternity Care, and Midwifery in North America and Europe.* Routledge, 2001.

[5] Tarkka, Marja-Terttu, et al. "Social Support Provided by Public Health Nurses and the Coping of First-Time Mothers with Child Care." *Public Health Nursing,* vol. 16, no. 2, 1999, pp. 114–119., doi:10.1046/j.1525-1446.1999.00114.x.

week postpartum checkup and the weeks and months following in which women are left to figure things out on their own.

Educating and empowering women is my passion. I want to give women the tools they need to live their best life free of physical ailments because, really, you only have one body; why not make it perform at its most optimal state?

"Who do I reach out to for help?" OR "Is there hope for me?" are common questions I get asked. Women are embarrassed and/or frustrated, and that often leads them down a road of feeling helpless and googling their symptoms to find a solution. Spending the past eight plus years of my life going through a number of specialized courses, studying and consulting with expert physical therapists in this field, and experiencing my own healing journey, I am ready to share with the world what has worked tremendously for me and the thousands of clients I have helped. I am excited for you to dive in and learn more, so thank you for taking the time to do so in the upcoming chapters.

Moms, you won't want to miss out on some bonus information at the book's conclusion; it just may change your life.

CHAPTER 1

THE REAL TRUTH
4 Common Mom Body Myths

Women face constant pressure to look like their pre-pregnancy selves so quickly after they deliver. As busy moms, we dismiss the fact that we need to focus on taking care of our bodies and allow them to heal properly; after all, it did take nine months to go through these changes. At the gym after a fitness class, I heard these following statements while listening to women discuss their postpartum body issues, and I will address each one so women can learn the truth!

1. *"I had a baby, so I'm going to have to deal with peeing when I cough, run, or jump."*

FALSE: This problem is definitely a common one, but no matter how long after you have a baby, it can continue to be an issue if not addressed. **Women dismiss this problem as something they are going to just have to deal with forever.** *Little do they know it can be assessed and treated rather quickly with the right guidance from a women's health PT.*

The issue is usually coordination and timing between breathing and the ability to contract the pelvic floor muscles. Pelvic floor muscle weakness and lack of endurance may exist as well just like any other muscles in the body. You don't have to "just-in-case pee" before you try to run because this can be fixed!

(More about this in the coming chapters)

2. "I can jump back into my old fitness routine because I feel fine."

FALSE: Many women who exercise during their pregnancy can ease back into their fitness routine feeling ok, but be forewarned, nine months of changes to your body don't automatically go back without the proper amount of time needed to heal. Your pelvis will be recovering and returning to a "pre-labor" state zero to six weeks postpartum, your uterus is contracting back to its previous state, and your internal organs are returning to their rightful place after being squished out of the way during pregnancy.

*Any intense activity during this stage could hinder the healing process. Jumping back into that boot camp class right after your six-week checkup may not be the best for all women as abdominal separation and pelvic floor weakness **are not assessed by all** OB/GYNs or **midwives**. These issues can lead to pelvic organ prolapse, a worsening of diastasis recti (abdominal separation), or back pain if you ramp up your program without proper guidance.*

Be your own advocate and seek out guidance from a PT who specializes in women's health issues; feel free to jump ahead to the chapter covering key exercises to consider first. It's very encouraging to have a professional who will not only provide you with the best exercises to promote healing, but will also set you up for success with high intensity exercise. Add gentle stretching, light resistance training, and walking to set you up for success in the early stages postpartum.

3. "My abdominals will get toned with lots of crunches."

FALSE: This is not always the case. Because your deeper layer of abdominals (transverse abdominis) has been stretched for the last nine plus months, it is important to train the abdominals from "the inside out." Crunches work the rectus abdominis (outer layer) and place unnecessary stress on the spine and pelvic floor without training the "inner core" first. **That doesn't mean you can never do crunches; it just means you need specific exercises to heal the inner layer first.**

Also, as I have mentioned earlier in this chapter, something called diastasis recti is very common where the abdominals actually separate during pregnancy, creating a disruption in the connective tissue layer below. In some cases, this heals itself naturally postpartum, but **it's very common for it to continue to be an issue three to six months (and beyond) postpartum.** *This may be why a woman feels like she just can't get rid of her abdominal "pooch" even though she is exercising and losing weight.*

I can't stress enough the importance of receiving an individualized assessment from a women's health PT who will prescribe specific exercises to your routine to help heal diastasis recti, which will avoid the need for surgery! (I have devoted an entire chapter to this topic!)

4. "My back pain will go away eventually."

FALSE: You could be experiencing back pain due to several reasons. The extra hormones that are released during pregnancy remain in your system up to four months after you stop nursing; this will affect the stability in your pelvis and joints. Lack of core strength and muscle imbalances, now that you aren't carrying another human inside of you, will affect the pressure placed on your back when lifting and carrying a baby car seat, stroller, heavy diaper bag, etc.! A proper strength training routine and practicing good body mechanics when lifting, holding, and caring for your baby will make a huge difference in your symptoms.

*Going through pregnancy and labor is a huge feat for a woman, and **it is important to be your own advocate if you are having these musculoskeletal issues that won't go away.***

In our practice, a Pilates-based approach to improving core and pelvic floor function is the best approach to building a strong foundation, allowing you to return to all those other fitness activities without back pain.

So, if something doesn't feel quite right, or you have been dealing with pain and other bothersome symptoms for too long, just know these myths after childbirth are just that...MYTHS!

CHAPTER 2

WOMEN'S HEALTH

What's the Pelvic Floor Got to Do with It?

Maybe you wear black yoga pants when working out to hide the embarrassing leaking that happens with jumping jacks or running. Or, maybe you came down with the flu, and your non-stop coughing made you uncontrollably leak so you had to wear a pad. Maybe just thinking about having sex again without pain seems like something in the distant past. Maybe the pressure you feel in your vaginal area when walking around is a little scary, and you're not sure if things are "in the right place" post-pregnancy. Maybe things feel "not quite right"—but you've just learned to deal with it for years.

Trust me, I have heard all of these situations in my office before and you are NOT alone.

*Are you a mom that is dealing with an issue you just assumed was a normal byproduct of childbirth? You're not the only one, and **I wrote this book because so many moms were telling me the same thing— "I didn't know you could fix this!"***

Many women have never heard of a pelvic floor PT. And doctors, instead of referring patients to someone like me, often may prescribe a medication, suggest surgery, or, even better, tell patients to "just give it some time and see if it gets better." Well, that just isn't good enough!

A PT is a musculoskeletal expert who helps people recover from an injury by using hands-on techniques like soft tissue work, joint manipulations, and exercise-based treatment to help correct faulty movement patterns and maximize their overall quality of life for the activities they want to do. While not *all* PTs address an entire muscle system called the "pelvic floor," they know about it, and would need further specialized training in how to properly assess and treat it!

Going to PT school, I got two hours of lecture in my entire graduate school experience on the "pelvic floor." Not to bore you with the details, but I realized after having my own babies that pelvic floor issues are absurdly COMMON, and there is an entire muscle system related to overcoming these embarrassing and frustrating issues. Medical doctors don't study the muscle systems as much as PTs do, even though they can be the source of so many issues like bladder leakage (called incontinence), painful sex, prolapse (or feeling of pressure in the pelvic region), birth-related trauma, and many other diagnoses related to the actual muscle system of the pelvic floor.

Not only that, but, often, undiagnosed back and hip pain can be related to a pelvic floor issue. Some PTs might take weeks trying to help resolve an ongoing chronic issue that actually could be related to a deeper problem within the pelvic muscle area, which affects mobility and stability of the hips/pelvis.

It's also important to add that women who have gone through menopause will experience atrophy (or weakening) in their pelvic floor muscles, thereby affecting bladder function and increasing the risk for pelvic organ prolapse due to the drop in estrogen levels. Many times, this leads to surgery for a prolapsed bladder (will get into this more in a future chapter), but if women were taught the principles in this book within the first six months after labor and delivery, I believe it could lead to a lot less of these post-menopausal issues. Women 30 years ago did not have the resources we have today; pelvic floor PT was extremely rare, and fitness was not as popular as it is today.

I think it is best practice to have ALL women do a postpartum check up with a pelvic floor PT, but AT LEAST at the six-week postpartum checkup, it should be included as part of a comprehensive assessment addressing issues that affect a woman's ability to go back to her prior activities.

OB/GYNs are not spending the time to address if your pelvic floor is weak, if your abdominals have separated (diastasis recti), or if you are at risk for prolapse like a pelvic floor PT would. But they DO say, "You are good to go back and exercise; your incision is healed," or "Everything is fine; just ease back into your old routine," without really knowing if your pelvic floor can withstand the force of running and jumping. It makes me crazy when a woman without proper guidance jumps back into boot camp classes or decides she wants to lose her baby weight so she begins training for a half marathon.

Really? I was there, too; how badly did I just want to feel like my old self again? It's common to brush this off, and it's not until a woman is seriously struggling with a painful issue or a seriously embarrassing one that she finally decides to seek help (or just stop doing the activity altogether).

Part of my purpose is just to get more information out there on the topic of checking in with a pelvic floor PT. (You do not need an MD referral, ladies!) This could save you a major issue in the future; you can actually recover faster if you learn some new things about your body and even optimize your performance in your activity! Wait, what? I can run faster and feel stronger if I do this? YES! Countless times I have helped women who do high intensity interval training, heavy weight lifting, or run marathons, and if the center of your body (the core, we call it) is not at its full recovery and strength, you are at a much higher risk for pelvic organ prolapse or a back injury. Plus, (even more info to wake you up!) your performance in the activity will suffer, as well. This is the center of your body and your powerhouse for lifting, carrying, and moving in life and sports.

The manual labor of caring for a new infant is sometimes enough to make you feel beat up with poor nursing posture, lifting heavy car seat carriers in and out of the car, holding an infant on your chest all day long, and lifting a stroller in and out of a car. So then, added exercise activity to get back in shape—with a midsection and pelvis that aren't functioning the right way—will set you up for failure. I am all for exercising; however, I'd rather see you do things in the proper order to set your body up for success in the long term. When you are 50 or 60, you will thank me!

Oftentimes, these issues aren't addressed until the baby is much older because moms put their kids' needs before their own. I see this all the time. If guidance from a pelvic floor PT were actually part of the standard of care from the beginning, then most of these issues would not be problematic later in life.

Here is an example:

> *Sarah, a 37-year-old female, from Carlsbad, California, came to me with concerns about how her body was recovering at three months postpartum. She had been to her OB/GYN six weeks postpartum and expressed concerns about how her abdominals were separated down the middle; she saw a doming and bulging ridge running vertically down her middle when she got up out of bed every day, and she was fearing what that meant in the long run. She also felt pain around her incision site from an episiotomy, which had healed, but by no means did she want to try and have sex because she still had pain.*
>
> *Sarah was given a few tips on how to massage it and was told to "just wait and see how it goes." She wasn't pleased with this advice, and, instead, went online and started looking for other information about her symptoms. Her goals were to go back to running and an online circuit training program she did at home when her baby was napping, but she was scared about doing something that might make things worse. In the process, she came across my website and called me.*
>
> *Sarah was feeling confused about where to start to feel like herself again and feel more confident about her body. It was part of her life before to have a routine that felt good to her, and she needed that in her life again. We worked together to meet her goals and to have her successfully return to her prior fitness routine. We restored her abdominal strength the right way, which also enabled her to return to intimacy with her husband without pain. In the end, her confidence was renewed, and, she understood her body in a new way.*

I hear countless stories like this, some including trauma or other emotional stress that comes with the physical issue they are experiencing. But time and time again, the commonality is the fact that a woman's life is being affected by the physical aspect of the condition, which causes even more worry and frustration. Maybe it is the area where I live (Southern California), but increasingly more information is available now that our mothers and grandmothers did not have. Some doctors are recommending a pelvic floor specialist, and also, with social media and recent press on NPR and mainstream news outlets, women are discovering more about these other resources that can help them.

What is the pelvic floor, and why do I need to know this?
(Trust me you need to understand this first)

The Pelvis and Pelvic Floor

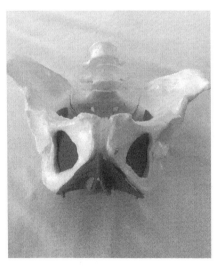 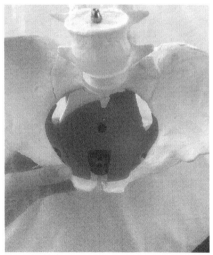

It can be thought of like a basket of muscles in the bottom part of your pelvis.

These layers stretch like a hammock from the tailbone at the back, to the pubic bone in front. A woman's pelvic floor muscles support her bladder, womb (uterus) and bowel (colon). The urine tube (front passage), the vagina, and the back passage all pass through the pelvic floor muscles. Your pelvic floor muscles help you to control your bladder and bowel; they also help sexual function.

The pelvic floor is a muscle system that should be called upon to work as much as necessary but as little as possible. It is a muscle system that is not trained like your biceps but more like a gauge for control and stability. Subconsciously your pelvic floor needs to fire when it's called upon, and is always in a state of protection and support for your pelvic organs. It's the key to bladder control—hence those embarrassing trampoline moments!

When we think of the "core" muscles, which go through significant change as they are stretched and stressed during pregnancy and delivery, we think of the pelvic floor as the bottom portion of the "core." The diaphragm controlling your breathing is at the top, the deep abdominal muscles in the front, and the multifidus (back stabilizing muscles) in the back portion. There are a ton of other muscles fully involved in controlling the movement of the middle of your body, but for the purposes of this book, I will be discussing the pelvic floor function as I address the aforementioned COMMON—but not normal—symptoms. Sadly, I find that women often just live with the physical problems and fail to seek out proper treatment.

Pelvic floor issues don't always just happen because of vaginal delivery with childbirth; they can be common even after a C-section or abdominal surgery.

Oftentimes, too, before a woman gets pregnant, she will display some symptoms of incontinence (leaking) with exercise or have painful sex, both issues that were never treated but now need to be addressed.

What gets women through the door at my office is the new realization that labor and delivery put obvious stress on the pelvic floor, which then needs to be re-trained. The symptoms prior to pregnancy were most likely due to an inability to actually relax and let go of those muscles. Yes, you might NOT need Kegel exercises! They can actually create the painful symptoms due to prolonged muscle holding patterns. But how would you know? Women usually aren't asked by their doctor, or maybe they have pain with a gynecological exam and were told to "just relax." But what if their muscles don't know how to relax? Yes, that is a thing. It's different with muscles like your biceps that have a voluntary ability to bend and straighten the elbow, but your pelvic floor is on autopilot, and, at times, needs to be taught how to actually relax and contract properly.

When you have a pelvic floor that is more restricted like this (difficulty with the relaxation portion), oftentimes the symptom can be described as "pain with intercourse." Women are often feeling anxiety about being intimate with their partner and are not enjoying sex because of uncomfortable pain. When this is the case, many of these women will have a lengthier labor process due to tighter pelvic floor muscles, and they don't even know that is the case. It's important for women to know it is not normal to have pain with sex or use of a tampon, and it can be relieved with the correct treatment strategy. As with any other muscle group in the body, the pelvic floor needs proper care.

A tear in the muscle during childbirth can cause an *overactive* pelvic floor. The tear may cause certain muscles to work too hard or become tight because they're tensing around tender spots. Some women develop an *overactive pelvic floor because they try to keep their pelvic floor muscles tensed for long periods.*

If you have tight muscles, you may continue to feel pain, even after your wound has healed. If you have an overactive pelvic floor, or very tight muscles, helpful treatment from a pelvic floor PT can provide trigger point massage, or trigger point release, as it's sometimes called.

Women are not guided properly through the steps of what to do to care for their postpartum self with a standard of care. Keep reading to find out what these steps are!

CHAPTER 3

POSTPARTUM

Timeline for Returning to Exercise

Here's a story to share with you...

> *Joanna, a 43-year-old female from Encinitas, California, came to me with concerns over her back pain. She was a new mom with a seven-week-old baby and had some new symptoms that were not present at her postpartum checkup two weeks ago. She began experiencing piercing back pain that radiated down to her buttock and hip when she bent over to pick up her child, which scared her as it had never happened before.*

> *Joanna also experienced increased pressure in the vaginal area while walking, and she had an increased urgency to get to the bathroom every time she needed to urinate. She searched online for clues about her symptoms, and that led her to seek out my help. It turned out she had a mild Stage 1 uterine prolapse and the beginning stages of a disc bulge, which was important to address sooner than rather so it didn't turn into a full-on herniation.*

I assessed her prolapse with a pelvic floor evaluation and instructed her to use specific strategies of breath work and proper Kegel technique to reduce the symptoms and improve her pelvic floor function. She learned how she should be lifting her baby and the car seat carrier, and I gave her targeted exercises to strengthen her trunk and hips in order to reduce strain on her spine. Within four visits she was feeling significantly better, less fearful, and more confident in her ability to control and improve her symptoms.

This is just one case, but so many other women who don't necessarily have pain or concerns about new symptoms just want to feel good in their own skin again, and it's not about how hard you work to do so; rather, it's about working smarter to get lasting results, which you will see in the stages I describe in this chapter.

What are the secrets to having the best physical healing postpartum and loving your new body? Now that you aren't carrying a watermelon-size human inside of you anymore, what is supposed to happen?

The postpartum period places a variety of new stresses on your body, in addition to what you have gone through after labor and delivery. My goal with this timeline is to guide women in the most OPTIMAL way, but do note that every woman's healing process is going to be different. Also, it is important to note that no matter how long after you've had a baby, it is important to go back to STAGE 2 and move forward. If any part of your physical body is in pain or not feeling quite right, it is important to address that first with your doctor and with a pelvic floor PT who will be able to guide you in the right direction. With that said, this is a general timeline that works really well for my clients; it can prevent issues down the road, and it can help clients perform better physically, while improving overall *physical health in the first year and beyond postpartum (or even if you are wanting to have another baby in the future!).*

STAGE 1: one to four weeks postpartum—Let yourself have downtime (healing time) for the first four weeks. Let people help you adjust to life with the baby and truly allow yourself to REST and recover. This does not mean starting yoga or walking hills outside with the stroller; it means really resting. Focus on sleep, hydration, and nutrition in this phase.

STAGE 2: four to eight weeks postpartum—At this point, you will likely have had your postpartum check up with your medical provider. Once you are cleared, the best decision you could make is to check in with a pelvic floor PT. At this session you will be assessed and guided by the expert in muscle function for returning to activity. You will be assessed internally to see how your pelvic floor muscles are functioning (even if you had a C-section, this is important) and for pelvic organ prolapse (see later chapter on this). You will learn efficient ways to ward off neck and back pain while caring for a baby. Your pelvic floor PT will assess abdominal muscle activation and separation (commonly called diastasis recti) and give you the best advice about what exercises to focus on for restoring your core and pelvic floor. Breath work, pelvic floor contractions/relaxation, and posture exercises are usually the best to start in this stage.

This is not the time to return to weight lifting and running, yet. Swimming, gentle yoga, body weight restorative exercises, and walking are the best activities in this stage. Nutrition (collagen-rich foods, healthy fats, and lean proteins are important) plus hydration (at least half your bodyweight in kilograms of water) is so important in this phase. Consulting with a nutritionist will also help you save time and energy with efficient and effective meal prep ideas.

STAGE 3: nine to 12 weeks postpartum—At this point, women who have increased activity levels may experience more back aches/pains because abdominal and back strength is not yet optimal. Your body is now performing activities that tend to promote rounded shoulders and a forward head posture, such as breastfeeding, carrying a baby, and lifting a car seat. When are you actually reversing that posture and spending time on your stomach or opening the chest/shoulders to stretch the front of your shoulders?

This stage is all about finding strength in your body again; it's about building a new foundation in your pelvic floor and core to prevent pelvic organ prolapse and set yourself up for success with higher intensity exercise. Also, the hormones still not leveling off from pregnancy (especially if you are still nursing) will continue to promote joint laxity, thereby affecting your ligaments; this will put more stress/strain in different areas if strengthening exercises are not introduced in this phase. Continue with restorative work, and begin weight training, with hip and core strengthening being the most beneficial. Yoga, Pilates (with a postnatal specialist), swimming, weight training, and walking are best during this phase.

*STAGE 4: 13 weeks ON—Anyone who has had a baby is forever postpartum. I don't like this phase to end as we go through different phases in our lives as women. From our teen years to childbearing stage, to menopausal and post-menopausal, we continue making improvements in our health journey and pelvic floor/core health. More intense exercise may be added at this stage **once foundational strength has been achieved.** How do we know this?*

Try these two tests on yourself to see if your muscles are reacting the right way:

a. *Try doing a **jump test** for two minutes. Can you perform jumping jacks or jump rope for two minutes straight without symptoms of pain, leaking, or anything else that doesn't feel quite right?*

b. *The **cough test**: Place your hand over your navel while standing. Feel what happens to your abdominals when you do a fake cough. Does your stomach push out into your hand? What you should have happen is a drawing in or contraction of your "core" muscles when you cough or sneeze instead of pushing outward. This is a reflex that can be trained to have a normal functional pelvic floor and deep abdominal reaction. Your muscles should automatically tighten and draw in before a cough or sneeze, and, if they don't, you have some work to do.*

For my clients, I can give you the guidelines with an assessment to set you up for success to return to running and HIIT-type workouts. Well, how do you know you are ready for this? Have you consistently been working on hip and core work at least three times each week for the past six weeks free from any back or pelvic pain? In my office, I can more extensively assess a woman's readiness for return to high intensity exercise, but, as a general, rule my recommendations are as stated above. I treat this phase as ongoing no matter how long after you had a baby. You can incorporate its exercises as part of a circuit training regimen in my workouts (see next chapter); this will prevent prolapse and maintain a healthy spine and pelvis (plus it will keep your midsection more toned!).

Visit level4pt.com/beyond-9-months for an online program and a virtual option to guide you through this entire phase.

CHAPTER 4

RESTORATIVE EXERCISE

It's Not the Boring Stuff and Keep It in Your Routine Forever!

The secret to successfully training "like a mother" is using restorative postpartum exercises in a program that enhances recovery after pregnancy (no matter how fit you think you are!), reduces risk for pain, gets you stronger from the inside out, and helps tone your body more efficiently.

This is the program that my 50- to 60-year-old clients wish they had known about when they were younger so they could have avoided issues they are now being advised to address with surgery. In fact, a study from the Harvard Women's Health Watch found that a group of women performing pelvic floor training showed much greater improvements in prolapse, bladder, and bowel symptoms. Seventy-four percent felt less vaginal bulging or heaviness, compared with 31 percent in the control group. Severity of prolapse improved by one full stage in 19 percent of pelvic floor muscle trained participants, compared with eight percent of the control group. The exercisers also had greater improvements in pelvic floor muscle strength and endurance and in bladder and rectum position.[6]

No, this is not the boring stuff...this is the bread and butter! In order to return to high intensity exercise, these restorative practices need to be a consistent part of your daily program for a good six to eight weeks prior to running, CrossFit, or any other high intensity exercise program. Maybe you don't have a goal to be that active in fitness; but if you do plan for a future pregnancy, or if you are reaching menopausal stage next, this is ALL going to apply to you. Also, if you want to lose the postpartum "mommy pooch" and optimize your bladder and sexual function, then this should be an integral part of your movement for the day.

All exercises incorporate breath work as the diaphragm plays a huge role in function of the midsection of your body. During pregnancy, your diaphragm is pushed up into your ribcage, you lose rotation of your upper back due to a growing belly, your lower back is in a more excessive curve due to the weight in the front of your body, and the pelvis has angled forward. These changes in posture don't all of a sudden revert to your pre-pregnancy self after you've given birth. Additionally, we have to account for new stresses your postpartum body is encountering. Your joints are more lax due to the hormone levels affecting your ligaments (and will continue as long as you are still breastfeeding), making you more susceptible to injury if you were to lift heavy objects or run a half mile. At this stage, you are most susceptible to pelvic organ prolapse, which is controlled by the strength and pressure in your pelvic floor region. The goal

---

[6] Harvard Health Publishing. "In the Journals: Pelvic Floor Muscle Training Can Help Reverse Pelvic Organ Prolapse." Harvard Health, Jan. 2011, https://www.health.harvard.edu/womens-health/pelvic-floor-muscle-training-can-help-reverse-pelvic-organ-prolapse.

of restorative work is to minimize risk for damage and prepare you for success. It is NEVER too late to add these as part of your program.

As an example, the following exercises later in this chapter can be incorporated as soon as four to six weeks postpartum to help with the foundation of healing. They will maximize your performance as a mom lifting car seat carriers and strollers; reverse your nursing posture bad habits; help you avoid peeing your pants while sneezing; and prevent pelvic organ prolapse and pain postpartum! Plus, if you plan to run or exercise, the best way to feel closer toward getting in shape is by having a stronger and more solid "core" foundation!

I could go on and on, but it's not about the specifics of the exercises, it's more about the breathing and control of the pelvic floor when you are doing these movements. It is about improving the way the muscles of the pelvic floor respond to increased pressure, like when you cough, sneeze, lift something heavy, or jump. It's about being more aware of your body by telling your pelvic floor what to do without thinking about it and feeling the pelvic floor respond. That is what is going to help you feel like yourself again in the long run, and it is the secret to training the right way in these first months postpartum! Additionally, if you are months or years later reading this, it is never too late to work on these exercises for enhanced support of your pelvic floor, improved control of the pelvic floor muscles (like stopping the leaking!), toned abdominals, and reduced back pain.

It is a misconception to believe that restorative exercise is unnecessary, and here are some of the common myths I hear from women that perpetuate that belief:

MYTH #1: *"Restorative exercise is boring!"*

In fact, this is not the case when you do it with purpose and even with your baby. Yes, it is possible to include your child in specific floor or standing exercises. Actually, it is more effective this way. Another fun way is to create a circuit of a 20-minute workout that will still get your heart rate up and make you break a sweat again (I totally forgot that feeling during my pregnancy!). You could perform four consecutive strengthening/restorative exercises with 10 to15 reps each; then add three to four minutes of pushing a stroller uphill while walking; do step ups on a small box/step, or alternate from sitting to standing from a park bench for 30 seconds in between the three rounds of exercises. This routine is not high-impact, but it is effective in burning calories, increasing your strength, and in being intentional about the exercises to get the benefits.

MYTH #2: *"I'm too tired."*

Ladies, this was my go-to. I was exhausted--but you know what? If I got myself to move for 20 minutes in the first part of the day, my mood changed immensely. In fact, exercise is shown to be the #1 most important intervention to improve postpartum depression and anxiety[7]; movement combined with proper nutrition during the early postpartum months can be a game changer.

---

[7] *Nakamura, Aurélie, et al. "Physical Activity during Pregnancy and Postpartum Depression: Systematic Review and Meta-Analysis." Journal of Affective Disorders, vol. 246, 2019, pp. 29–41., doi:10.1016/j.jad.2018.12.009.*

MYTH #3: "I don't know what I should be doing because I'm scared."

First of all, don't go on YouTube or Google to find "postnatal fitness" routines or an exercise plan. Not a good idea. You need guided expertise for YOUR individual needs. This is where a specialist comes into play. Don't know how to find one in your town? Then use Google and search "pelvic floor physical therapy near me." If you are in a remote area or still unsure of where to find the right PT (especially one who also has a fitness specialty), then check out this page: *level4pt.com/beyond-9-months/*

Or, if you are local Southern California, visit: *level4pt.com/womens-health* to set up a phone call with one of our women's health specialists to find out more!

This is the backbone of training for moms—no matter where you are in life—and, most importantly, it will help you regain internal confidence in your body and what it was made for!

These exercises start with proper breathing as the foundation, which can be integrated later into lifting weights and your baby, and into any other strenuous task that increases stress on your abdominals and pelvic floor.

Proper breathing is incredibly important for healthy pelvic floor function. Our primary breathing muscle is the diaphragm, a dome-shaped muscle that operates like a parachute. It connects to the lower part of the ribcage. The intercostals, little muscles that fit between your ribs, also play a primary role in breathing. These secondary breathing muscles, known as scalenes, are located in front of the neck, the pectoralis in the chest, the sternocleidomastoid from behind the ear to the sternum, and the upper trapezius.

Let's take another look at the diaphragm. When we bring in air from the mouth or nose, the lungs expand and the diaphragm muscle moves down toward the pelvic floor. So, on the inhalation, the diaphragm pushes our organs down into a sack called the peritoneum. And where does that sack of muscles get pushed? To the pelvic floor.

This is why breath is such an important part of pelvic floor work. When we breathe in, the pelvic floor is receiving the breath and the downward-moving organs. As we exhale, the breath goes up and out. The organs also move up. A healthy pelvic floor stretches as we breathe in *and* contracts slightly as the breath goes up and out.

Connecting it all together

We've looked at the connection between the diaphragm and the pelvic floor. But there's another key player in the healthy function of the pelvic floor: our abdominals.

Particularly important is the transverse abdominis, the deepest abdominal muscle, which is like a corset that goes all the way around the lower torso, attaching at the bottom ribs. The fibers of the transverse abdominis are horizontal, which means when they're contracted, they pull in the diameter of the abdomen (imagine tightening a belt). These muscles also serve a purpose in exhaling the breath.

If we have "poor" posture or spend a lot of time sitting in chairs, our transverse abdominis muscle will be weak. This, in turn, can be linked to pelvic floor problems. For example, if we collapse our chest while sitting, we end up with a "C-curve" in the spine. This makes it challenging to take a deep breath, and as a consequence, the muscles of the pelvic floor don't receive the gentle "exercise" they need of stretching and contracting with every breath in and out.

In short, if our posture is not good and we're not taking in deep breaths to the abdomen, our pelvic floor is most definitely suffering. Everything is connected, and deep belly breathing is the most efficient way to take care of the pelvic floor.

It's not easy to change breathing habits and patterns, and the key is never to force. But to get you started on deepening the breath, here's a little exercise you can try.

Deepening the breath:

1. *Lie on your back with knees bent and feet hip width apart.*

2. *To begin, take a few minutes to tune in to your body. Notice how you're feeling; notice areas with tension or tightness. Notice the movement of the breath, not judging or trying to change anything, just observing.*

3. *Put one hand on your lower belly below the navel, the other on your chest. Allow yourself to feel the breath move under your hands for a couple of minutes.*

4. *Then, as you exhale, gently contract the lower abdomen, moving the navel toward the spine. Repeat a few times, each time emptying out the air more fully. As you inhale, let the belly relax and soften. Allow the air to fill your lungs as the belly naturally inflates. Repeat three to five breaths; then just relax and return to your normal breath. Rest.*

5. *For round two, again draw the navel toward the spine as you exhale. As you get used to adding the sighing sound on the exhale, begin to add it on a small inhale as well; this will challenge the diaphragm and make the movement of the breath slightly deeper. Repeat this breath eight to ten times or as long as comfortable; then again, relax and return to your normal breath.*

Doing this simple breath exercise a couple of times a day or at the start of the day will go a long way toward strengthening and engaging the diaphragm, and, in turn, it will slowly deepen your breath over time.

Next...more of the action steps!

MY FANTASTIC 5 POSTNATAL FAVORITE EXERCISES:

(for pelvic floor and abdominal engagement...does not include the mobilty exercises I commonly give too)

Try these movements and incorporate them daily, even with your baby:

I. ***Diaphragmatic breathing:*** *(more detailed above) Position yourself on your back with knees bent; keep the shoulders and neck relaxed. Inhale through the nose and exhale through the mouth, allowing the rib cage to expand side to side and the belly to rise. Imagine the air flowing all the way down into your pelvis as you inhale and the ribs expanding like an umbrella opening and closing. Repeat for one to two minutes focusing on the breath going into your torso and all the way down below your navel.*

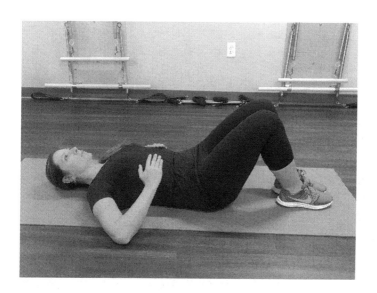

2. ***Pelvic floor activation with breathing:*** *Next, add the breathing with the pelvic floor activation by inhaling as in the first exercise, keeping the body relaxed. Upon exhale, imagine yourself stopping the flow of urine and stopping yourself from passing gas by bringing the urethra and the anus together on the exhale. Another cue that has worked well in my practice is imagining holding a blueberry in your vaginal area and lifting that blueberry up on your exhale only. So, you stay relaxed on the inhale and exhale with the pelvic floor muscle lift. Repeat 10-15 times, five times a day in this position, then in standing or sitting. DO NOT PERFORM pelvic floor exercises while sitting on the toilet; this will confuse your muscles and interrupt healthy bladder habits.*

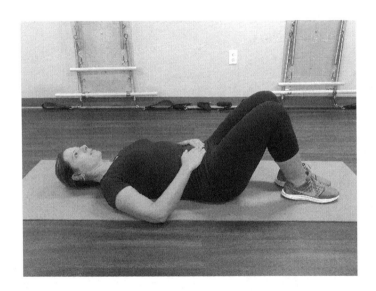

(See Chapter 10 on more pelvic floor activation steps.)

3. ***Bridging with pelvic floor activation:*** This exercise will be just like #2, but on your exhale and pelvic floor contraction, you will lift your hips up like a bridge exercise while adding a gluteal (butt) squeeze. Engage the pelvic floor and glutes on the exhale, and inhale as you lower your hips. Don't let your ribs flare out when you lift and keep the connection of the pelvic floor drawing in as you lift and bring navel to the spine. Repeat 10-15 times, three sets.

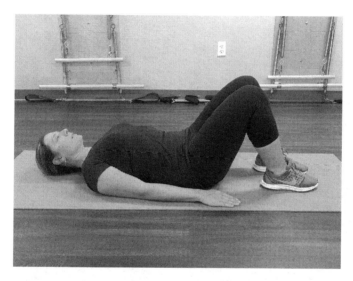

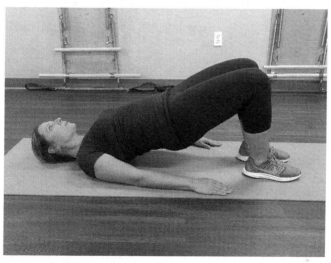

4. ***Squats with breath work:*** Here is one of my favorites because it encourages a functional movement you do throughout the day anyway! Perform in front of a chair or a box by standing on the exhale and inhale as you sit back down. You will engage your pelvic floor, glutes, and lower abdominals upon standing and during the exhale. To coordinate this exercise may take a few days, but keep practicing to train your brain to connect to the pelvic floor and core muscles again!

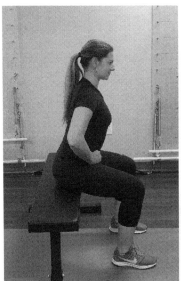 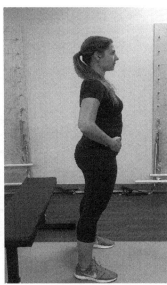

5. ***Wall angels for posture:*** *This one I added to the list to reverse the rounded shoulders and forward head posture we spend so much time in as moms while holding or nursing babies. The scapular (upper back/shoulder muscles) are meant to activate through the full range of motion. Plus, it also helps as a great exercise if you find yourself at a computer or hunched over a desk for long hours. For this exercise, keep your upper back against the wall and step out with your feet.*

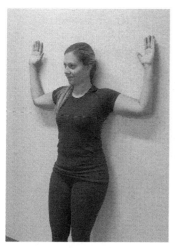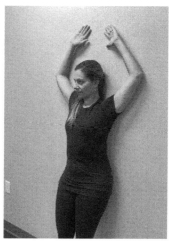

The upper back stays in contact with the wall, and arms will be out at a 90-degree angle from the shoulders. Maintain elbows and forearms against the wall while sliding your arms up and down as if making a snow angel. (Yes, I grew up in Ohio in the snow!) Repeat ten times sliding up and down, feeling the shoulder blades moving and upper back muscles engaging. If you can't maintain your arms against the wall, you probably have really tight chest and shoulder muscles, so modify this exercise by keeping at least your elbows against the wall. (You may need to see a PT if you are having shoulder or neck pain and you are that tight!)

6. ***Deadlifts with car seat carrier (or a weight)*:** *You are doing this already, aren't you—lugging the car seat carrier from car to house or store to car because you don't want to disturb your sleeping baby, right?*

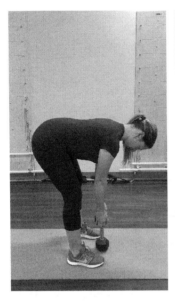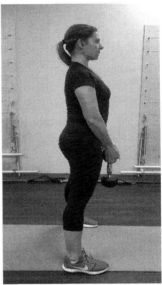

You need to incorporate proper breathing and engage the right muscles in these lifting mechanics so you keep your back and pelvic floor healthy. Place your hands on the sides at the top and bottom of the carrier (or a kettlebell/dumbbell) as pictured. Bend from the hips (not your back!) and exhale with the lift, engaging your pelvic floor, abdominals, and glutes on the way up. Inhale, but don't fully let go of your muscles as you lower the car seat carrier. Repeat with baby inside keeping the carrier close to your body as much as possible to avoid using your back. This is more of a hip exercise and a healthy one for your back if you are doing it correctly. Your back should not round! You should bend from the hips with a slight bend

in the knee. Repeat ten times, perform three sets, and don't forget to breathe!

The purpose of these exercises is to start integrating your breathing with your pelvic floor in order to encourage healthy habits when caring for your children and performing all the active things we do as moms in life! Use these as "go-to" exercises throughout motherhood!

CHAPTER 5

DIASTASIS RECTI

What Happened to My Abs?

One of the most common issues I see in my practice of treating women after pregnancy is diastasis recti (or abdominal separation). This condition is a lot more common than women think and has garnered more hype over the past few years. The extra weight some women carry around the midsection after delivering a baby can be confused with true diastasis recti. As you read on, you can learn more about deciphering the difference. You still look and feel four to five months pregnant even though it's been months or years since you delivered your baby; or, you see the line in the middle of your abs bulge outward when you go to sit up. Is this really a problem? At times when women think they have a diastasis, they read information online or hear horror stories from friends, which leads to avoidance of core and abdominal exercises because they are told these will make their condition worse.

Almost 100 percent of women have this condition during the third trimester of pregnancy; the belly button turns into an "outie," and when sitting up in the morning to get out of bed, the belly pooches out with a pronounced ridge upon exertion to standing. Truth be told, this separation is extremely

47

common, but if it is still present after eight weeks postpartum, it very well might be true diastasis recti.

What is diastasis recti?

This can be described by a thinning of the linea alba or connective tissue that lies between the superficial layer of your rectus abdominis (the six-pack ab muscles). This results in what looks like a separation between the superficial muscle; it can be measured by how many fingers can fit in the space. It's important to consider not only the width, but also the depth of a finger in the space, which is even more important. Also, if this is assessed by a medical professional, then a movement and strength assessment is even more beneficial to determine if it is going to be a problem or not.

Most women seek help for a diastasis in my practice because they fear it will worsen; they are concerned about not feeling like they used to when they return to doing specific ab/core exercises; they hate how it looks and want to feel good in their own skin again; or they plan to have another baby in the future and fear it will only get worse. For all these previous reasons, we come to terms, and I help them decide their most important reason for seeking help; what can be done about it; an approximate time frame it will take to improve; and how to keep active and prevent it from getting worse while carrying out daily tasks and caring for their family.

Avoiding an invasive surgery is definitely optimal, but some severe cases (over five finger widths of a separation at the midline) may eventually require surgery. You don't truly know until you seek out the conservative methods first, finding a PT that specializes in treating this. For some women, however, they are told surgery is the *only* option to "fix" it. This is absolutely false. In some cases, surgery MAY be an option, but it is definitely not the first option. I even asked my own OB/GYN six weeks *after having my 9 lb. 2 oz. baby what he would tell his patients (by the way he never assessed this on me. I had to ask, and he didn't even do it correctly. lol). He said, "Well, the only way to change that is surgically." He almost fell out of his chair when I told him that as a pelvic floor (and postnatal specialist) PT, I treat this all the time, and there are specific exercises and hands-on techniques to speed up the healing process. That just goes to show that misinformation that exists among ladies who have only sought advice from one medical practitioner.*

Self-check time

Check out this video to perform your own self-assessment. Check out the video on our YouTube Channel (LEVEL4 Physio) and click "Diastasis Recti Self-Assessment."

Why is diastasis recti a concern?

Many women are concerned about diastasis recti for aesthetic reasons. I hear, "Will my abs ever go back to normal?" Some say, "I've lost the baby weight, but I still have a bulge at my abdominal area that won't go away."

Women also fear activities they have heard (too much Google searching) may make it worse like certain yoga poses, sit-ups, planks, or twisting activities. Women tell me they don't feel confident in doing an effective workout in a fitness class. Additionally, they fear having another baby might make it worse. This might be true, but it might not be; as I say, it completely depends on the individual!

Interestingly enough, with women who seek help for diastasis recti, we find additional issues may be present. Postnatal back pain or stress incontinence (leaking urine with coughing, sneezing, and activity) may exist with diastasis recti, although research does not link them together. I have found that when we solve one issue, the other improves significantly, as well. The muscle system links all of these issues together, and my methods for improving a diastasis include the entire pelvis, hips, back and abdominals as a complementary unit that works together. It is NOT just about your abdominals, and no matter how many YouTube videos you find on "diastasis exercises" or "postnatal exercises," you are going to get the BEST outcome by working directly with a pelvic floor PT.

How is the "core" connected?

Because the abdominals are really just one portion of the "core," here is why I say it is a full system that can tone your midsection even better! The anatomy of your "core" makes up your diaphragm for your breathing at the top. The sides and front are your transverse abdominis (deepest abdominal layer). The pelvic floor makes up the bottom (like a basket of muscles that support your pelvic organs). And your multifidus is your stabilizing muscle along your spine in the back. A whole slew of other muscles and fascia connect to your spine, ribs, and pelvis, which impact the function of your midsection. When the abdominals are lacking strength, the other aspects of your trunk and pelvis will not function as a true efficient system.

What do I need to do to fix it?

The first step is going to my YouTube channel (LEVEL4 Physio) and type in "Diastasis Recti –Core Foundations Series" and start those exercises repeating at least ten reps each side for the series. It will talk you through the breath work with the leg movements to learn how to actually control your deep abdominal muscles. If this is difficult for you, or you are consistently working on these daily for a few weeks and feel no change, or you see a raised ridge down the center of your midsection when you try the exercises, then you need to seek out help of a highly skilled pelvic floor PT that has experience with treating diastasis recti (not a general PT).

Pelvic floor dysfunction with "leaking" and back pain won't eventually fix itself; neither will diastasis recti. They will require skilled intervention to resume that firing connection between the brain and the muscular system; this is called neuromuscular training.

For some women, it may even take a pelvic floor assessment and proper instruction in how to activate the deep layer of muscles with hands-on techniques. Sometimes the fascia from the lower back can be released to improve the activation of the muscles in the front of the body. This skilled intervention by a pelvic floor PT specialist may include techniques to optimize the length of tight or shortened muscles that won't cooperate with exercises alone.

This is why continuing to modify your workouts around diastasis recti will only get you so far. Your "core" is a term for a true muscular system that needs to work efficiently to reduce injury, improve your performance (especially for sports and running), and optimize pelvic health in relation to sexual function and bladder control. It's also important for preventing long-term problems from leading to surgery in the future (a whole different chapter coming later on pelvic organ prolapse!). For now, get assessed by a pelvic floor and/or women's health PT if you are concerned about this issue. Your body will thank you!

What to do next?

If you want to find out information on other natural, holistic options, click the link to get your free tips guide (level4pt.com/diastasis-recti), or if you live out of the area, we can schedule a call to guide you in the right direction.

CHAPTER 6

POSTURE AND PILATES

The First Change to Help Diastasis Recti and Pelvic Floor Health

A big part of my training and my practice focuses on Pilates and using the principles of Pilates to encourage healthy posture with stability and mobility of the spine. Pilates instruction can vary from place to place depending on the instructor's training and style, but when taught by a rehab professional, it maximizes using the deep core muscles of the "powerhouse"–the abdominals, back, and pelvic floor–to support your posture and learn how it all integrates together to improve your performance in life (and your symptoms, if that is the case). The exercises and instruction serve the purpose of allowing the shoulders to relax, the neck and head to move freely, and of relieving stress on the hips, legs, and feet, all while using your pelvic floor and abdominals in sync with your breathing.

Alignment and posture are KEY elements for improving diastasis recti. For example, because your rib cage has expanded during pregnancy and is offset by positioning more in front (or anterior to) of your pelvis, it is going to create increased tension on your abdominal area. In order to improve the outward "pooch" in your abdominals, your goal would be to vertically position your ribs right over your pelvis. Creating a position to decrease the pressure in the intra-abdominal area is essential. You can't firm up the midline of your abs, nor can you solve other pressure-related problems (such as a pelvic organ prolapse, hernia, varicose veins, and hemorrhoids) without tackling the root cause.

Here are some steps you can take on your own to begin making some changes:

#1: CREATE LENGTH IN THE SPINE (GET "TALLER")

If you do yoga, you've probably heard this one before. It's a fantastic cue.

Imagine that you are adding space in between the vertebrae. Start at the bottom of the spine, and gently make your way up the spine, feeling that you're getting taller and taller until you make it all the way to the crown of the head.

This simple action may very well already make you feel lighter and more confident, and things may even seem a little less "heavy"—a morale-booster! (When our posture is slouchy, this actually weighs down onto the muscles of the spine as well as the organs in the torso, thus actually making us feel heavier!)

#2: "ELEVATOR" BREATHING

Once you've found length in your body, you add the breath.

This breathing exercise will help to bring the breath down into the belly so it can fill the entire body.

Start the inhale breath in your belly; then let it travel up the torso like an elevator, filling the rib cage, sides of the body, and finally the lungs. Exhale; come back down the "elevator," emptying the lungs, ribs, and belly.

Inhale: belly, rib cage, pelvic, and lungs fill up
Exhale: pelvis, lungs, rib cage, belly empty out

This is an excellent breathing tool in preparation for birth, too!

#3: OPEN YOUR CHEST

Roll the shoulders a few times, front to back; then do one last shoulder roll, forward, and up and back. **From there, very gently and lightly, let the shoulders release and drop themselves "onto" the rib cage, as naturally as you can. Your shoulders should feel more "open" or wider.**

Keep this "opening" action in the shoulders, and bring your breath into the space between the shoulder blades.

A simple way to perform this exercise is to visualize sticking your chest out just a bit.

Avoid squeezing the shoulder blades together.

* *This helps remove stress in the shoulder area.*
* *Still think of softening the front ribs downward to avoid pressing the rib cage out (or flaring the ribs), especially if you want to improve diastasis recti.*

#4: NOW USE THE ABDOMINALS AND PELVIC FLOOR THE RIGHT WAY!

Activating the pelvic floor and deep abdominal muscles will sustain and support the length in the spine that we are aiming for, and it is essential in prenatal health and postnatal recovery.

In regards to bettering our posture, engaging the pelvic floor will help to sustain the core musculature at the base of the torso.

You may notice that adding Kegels to your walk helps to generate an "uplifted" feeling to your body, while continuing to tone the lower body. To sustain good posture, a healthy and toned pelvic floor is essential.

* *Breath should remain steady.*
* *Incorporating movement to any Kegel work will help to integrate the pelvic floor exercises into the overall functionality of the body by creating connections and strengthening deep core muscles; this is what we're aiming for!*

I always teach women to integrate the pelvic floor (i.e., do Kegel first, and then pull the belly button in with your EXHALE):
Think of it this way:

1. *Slightly close and "lift" the pelvic floor (think of holding a blueberry in at your vaginal area and keep it lifted).*
2. *Pull the area below your belly button toward the spine very slightly; imagine the tips of the hips moving towards each other.*

*This will activate the transverse abdominal and "core" musculature, creating a kind of **corset of support around the spine**. It's a lovely way to* *feel supported, uplifted, and even a bit "lighter." (And it feels so good to finally feel the abs again when you're a postnatal mama.)*

#5: BRING YOUR RIB CAGE RIGHT OVER YOUR PELVIS

Bring your attention to the rib cage, which often will be positioned in front of the hips (almost like your ribs are flaring out), imagining that you want to align vertically the back of the head with the back of the pelvis.

The pull on your abdominals might feel greater when your rib cage is not aligned right over your hips. Think of growing taller and keeping those ribs right over your hips in standing or sitting, which creates less tension in the abdominal area, allowing you to breathe more freely. The position of your ribs does make a difference.

Notice if you are reverting to a pregnancy posture; *there might be a chance your butt is sticking out and you are flaring your ribs out. Try reducing the sway in the lower back by **slightly** tucking the tailbone forward (posterior tilt), and think of "knitting" the ribs together in front of your body to change your alignment.*

And, on the contrary, there might be *a chance your butt is tucked in. Try bringing a little bit more of the natural curve back into the lower back by **slightly** sticking the butt out (slightly!!) (anterior tilt).*

*   *The base of the chin should be more or less parallel to the ground.*
*   *Keep a slight bend in the knees to avoid hyperextension.*
*   *Relax the jaw.*

#6: DEEP BREATH RELEASE (OR A BIG "SIGH")

Sighing releases tension and invites us to breathe deeply. A full breath oxygenates the body, nourishing and helping to strengthen the postural muscles surrounding the spine.

It's also a great way to release tension in the body and mind.

#7: RELAX WHAT DOESN'T NEED TO BE "WORKING."

*You might also recognize this cue from yoga classes; it is another wonderful tip for good posture, **and also for finding focus and relieving stress in day-to-day life.***

What does this mean in my daily life?

You know how sometimes when you're working hard on something, you realize at one point that you're tensing up other parts of the body, say the forehead, jaw or shoulders, as if these parts of the body want to "work" with you?

Bring your attention to the feet and legs; although we're maintaining tone there, can the toes (for example) relax a bit more? Or maybe the hips?

Then see if the shoulders and jaw are relaxed.

And, finally, the facial muscles. Bring your gaze a bit further ahead of you, and think of relaxing all the "skin" of your face.

* *This helps to calm and focus the mind by bringing the attention back to the present moment.*
* *Keep breathing!*

By aiming at feeling the spine long and our body properly aligned, we can most definitely feel the effects on the mind, possibly bringing on a more positive, confident, and aware mind and body to support the center of your body and improve the appearance of your abdominals! To learn more about the benefits of Pilates or to even try a free session at our studio visit: level4pt.com/pilates.

CHAPTER 7

STRESS INCONTINENCE

Fear the Trampoline With Your Kids Because You Pee Your Pants?

Honestly, this is my favorite chapter. Know why? It is the most common misconception about life after kids, no matter if it's been weeks or YEARS! I often hear: "I will never be able to do that," OR "I just start peeing my pants so I don't do that," OR "Ever since I had kids, I can't do that." Having babies comes with its aftermath, for sure, but is peeing your pants something you just have to live with now?

This leakage issue is called "stress incontinence."

In fact, a study of 290 regularly exercising women revealed 47 percent incidence of urinary incontinence. Twenty percent stopped a routine exercise due to urinary incontinence, 18 percent modified routine exercise to avoid it, and 55 percent wore a pad during exercise...55 percent!!![8] The

---

[8] *Nygaard, Ingrid, et al. "Exercise and Incontinence." Obstetrics and Gynecology, vol. 75, no. 5, May 1990, pp. 848–851,*

researchers found that jumping, high impact landings, and running all promote urinary incontinence problems, hence the trampoline dilemma!

Client story:

> Cynthia is a 41-year-old mom with a 3-year-old. She came to me after a severe two-week bout with pneumonia where she suffered from intense coughing. Every time she had a coughing fit, she began to lose bladder control, and this was something new for her. She thought it was just a fluke because she was coughing so hard. As Cynthia recovered, she went to a playdate with her daughter who begged her to jump on a trampoline with her; but she began to lose bladder control again. It was enough to make her believe that she couldn't do that anymore because she couldn't control herself. Her friend laughed with her, saying the same thing happens to her so she doesn't go on it. It wasn't until later on when I met Cynthia at an event and gave a talk on pelvic floor and bladder control, that her ears perked up. She admitted to me later how embarrassed she was, and she wondered if she could fix it.

Cynthia's story is incredibly common. In fact, this is usually the top women's health issue that women do *not* seek help for because they do not know a PT can treat it. Doctors and women often discount incontinence as being a normal part of motherhood. Doctors will direct new mothers to do Kegel exercises after labor and delivery without any sort of follow up or direction; and other women will often say to new mothers that it "just happens after you have babies; join the club." I hear it in the women's restroom at the gym; I hear it when women are socializing; and I hear it

---

journals.lww.com/greenjournal/Abstract/1990/05000/Exercise_and_Incontinence.26.aspx #pdf-link.

from my friends. This is called stress incontinence, and many times it is a reflex that can be trained along with pelvic floor muscle control training.

First, it's important to keep track of any DYSFUNCTIONAL BLADDER HABITS you might have. Any of the following habits could lead to a long-term issue:

1. *"Just in case" peeing. You are anticipating that long car ride, you see the fitness routine that you are planning to do, or you see a bathroom prior to getting on an airplane and decide, "I should just go now before I really have to." Repetitive "just in case" peeing leads to dysfunctional habits and a programmed response for the bladder to empty even before it's full. This can lead to more urgency in the long run.*

2. *Semi-squatting on the toilet. In this case, please sit your entire bottom on the toilet. I don't care what you have to do to clean the toilet seat (wipe off the seat, use extra toilet paper on the seat, etc.), but if you semi-squat over the seat, you aren't fully emptying your bladder because your pelvic floor muscles can't completely relax.*

3. *Don't strain to pee. Pushing or forcing out urine also does not come from a place of full relaxation of the pelvic floor.*

4. *Don't do your Kegel exercises on the toilet. This will confuse your bladder and muscles. We use this as a cue to know which muscles you actually need to contract during a Kegel exercise, but please don't do it while sitting on the toilet; save it for other times during the day.*

Now, see what you are doing that is on the list for HEALTHY BLADDER HABITS:

1. *Sit all the way down on a toilet when you go to the bathroom. (Yes, I just repeated this from above). Sitting all the way down on the toilet will allow your bladder to empty completely.*

2. *Urinate every three to four hours on average.*

3. *Aim for an "8 Mississippi" count as a normal amount of time you should be actually peeing. If you are going a lot longer than that, then you are probably waiting too long to void. On the other hand, if it is markedly less time than that, then you are going too often and you have a high level of urgency. This could mean you need to do some bladder training, and try to see if you can train yourself to hold it an extra 15 to 20 minutes each time you get the urge.*

4. *Able to hold the need to urinate during the night and not wake up to pee. This habit is common after pregnancy because we were automatically trained to get up during the night because of the extra pressure on our bladder from the growing baby. After pregnancy, without the baby pressing against your bladder, you have gotten used to the habit, plus you might be up multiple times during the night, anyway, with nightly baby feedings.*

5. *Positioning when urinating. Keep a slight forward tilt in the pelvis with a straight spine. Don't curl your tailbone underneath you as this places more pressure on the pelvic organs and doesn't allow for full relaxation of the pelvic floor muscles.*

6. *Avoid constipation. Eating fiber in your diet and keeping ahead of any constipation symptoms can prevent you from over straining*

and having extra pressure on your pelvic floor, which can even impact bladder function.

7. *Go before or right after sex:* Urinary tract infections are unquestionably associated with sexual intercourse. Cystitis is common after sexual intercourse and is another word for inflammation of the bladder. One of the major reasons that intercourse is thought to be associated is that penetration can put pressure on the urethra. This can irritate the urethra or force bacteria up into the urethra and toward the bladder. In turn, this raises the likelihood of infection.

I want to share with you some causes of stress incontinence and also what you may be able to change on your own to see improvement. Pelvic floor PTs do treat this because it can be a muscle control issue.

Try these things on your own first:

1. **Diet/fluid intake habits:** Eliminate certain foods or drinks out of your diet, especially two hours before you exercise. Caffeinated beverages like coffee and tea, which sounds pretty obvious, can be stimulants to your bladder, and so they make your bladder feel full much more quickly and gives you the urge to eliminate. Also, drinks with artificial sweeteners, carbonation, highly acidic foods, or dairy products can also do the same. Cutting those out of your diet and seeing if that makes a difference may help.

2. **Work on breathing exercises:** Diaphragmatic breathing and getting in tune with your pelvic floor to release and let go prior to a Kegel exercise is just as important as the actual contraction. I have a video on my YouTube channel titled "Pelvic Floor Relaxation" that will teach you these exercises.

3. *Train your pelvic floor for the stress:* Think of squeezing a blueberry in your vaginal opening, and keep it there. While you hold it, try doing a fake cough. After the cough, release the imaginary blueberry. Repeat ten times; perform at least three to four times per day. This is training a reflex that normally should work to contract your pelvic floor before a sneeze or cough. Sometimes your pelvic floor is doing the opposite and pushing those muscles out, rather than "in and up," with a physically demanding effort or during a cough or sneeze. Try performing this action prior to lifting something heavy or lifting an object from the floor. It's like a "pre-set" contraction of your pelvic floor *before* you exert yourself.

Try doing these three things consistently and daily for the next three weeks. If you test it and you are still getting symptoms, then keep reading....

4. The next thing that I would address is making sure you're doing the *right* kind of exercises. I know many people would recommend, "Oh, just do your Kegel exercises." Well, **a lot of times that is not necessary, or it is, to a point, but you have to learn how to do them correctly.**

And if you're having these bladder issues, it could be because you have some internal muscle holding (like your muscles have trouble letting go), or the weakness or timing of your contractions needs some individualized guidance. Many times, women who see me don't even know if they are contracting the muscle correctly, or they engage their abdominals, inner thighs, and gluteal muscles all together to compensate.

A pelvic floor PT will guide you with a possible need for some internal massage work to release those tight muscles so you can generate a stronger contraction. A PT can also teach you how to do the appropriate exercises for the exact problem you are having (strength vs. endurance problem) and help you progress toward jumping or running as your pelvic floor learns what it is supposed to do. Bottom line: Stress incontinence is not going to fix itself, and you need some professional guidance. The muscles that help support your bladder and other pelvic organs have to be taught the right way to function again after nine months of increased pressure and from the stress of labor and delivery.

So, I just wanted you to know that this is a common issue, and it can be treated. Working on the right strengthening exercises with a professional as a guide can really do wonders for your body; sometimes it's a quick fix, too!

Now, when you are jumping or running and you begin "leaking" after just a few seconds or minutes, you may have a problem with your strength or endurance. Training Kegel contractions first in static positions, then gradually increasing the intensity with functional movements like squats, low impact jumping jacks, or bounding activities can be an excellent and successful way to train your body the way it is meant to function.

A variety of reasons exist for why this problem occurs only with exertion. If this only seemed to be an issue after pregnancy, it could be that the neural pathway to your muscles got confused or interrupted after you were conditioned to get up and pee frequently because of the pressure the baby placed on your pelvic floor during pregnancy. It just needs the right type of training again. Or, this is truly a weakness issue and your pelvic floor muscles can't sustain the graded contraction when an impact or increased force is placed upon them; therefore, strengthening in the right manner and progression can be hugely successful.[9]

Like I mentioned before, if your muscles do hold extra tension and you can't tell the difference between relaxing and contracting, then when you jump or run the muscles are not going to be able to respond to the stress in the most optimal manner, and you may need some professional guidance. The bottom line is that you can stop being embarrassed and quit using a pad or dark colored yoga pants on that next workout if you get this fixed!

For more incontinence tips like this, please visit this special information website: *level4pt.com/stress-incontinence. You'll find a free 15-page guide waiting for you that shows you six more amazing tips to stop the embarrassment of "leaking" with sneezing or exercise! (A Women's Guide to Improve Symptoms of Stress Incontinence).*

The next few sections relate to issues that can stop you during pregnancy and is the most common issue I treat as well, so read on, ladies!

---

[9] *Cavkaytar, S., et al. "Effect of Home-Based Kegel Exercises on Quality of Life in Women with Stress and Mixed Urinary Incontinence." Journal of Obstetrics and Gynaecology, vol. 35, no. 4, 2014, pp. 407–407, doi:10.3109/01443615.2014.960831.*

CHAPTER 8

BACK PAIN

How to Defeat This Frustrating Problem That Hinders You from Staying Active

As a busy mother, nothing can be more frustrating than the aches and pains from postnatal back pain that slow you down. Lifting your kids into a crib or car seat, pushing a stroller, chasing your kids through the store when they try running away, or carrying a heavy diaper bag all put extra strain on your back. If you haven't fully recovered from labor and delivery, or it's been months (or even years!) and you aren't feeling your best, then read on; there are solutions to help you.

Back pain after labor has many causes, but two of the main causes are posture changes and hormonal changes.

Posture can change during pregnancy as the weight of the baby during the last trimester shifts the pelvis forward and increases the curve in the lower back. This can lead to postnatal back pain if your abdominal muscles are still weak, but you are still in a habitual pregnancy posture; most of that stress still goes to your back.

Hormonal changes can also contribute to back pain. The production of Relaxin during pregnancy and beyond (even when you are nursing) increases the laxity in your joints and may continue to be in your body for up to six months after you stop nursing. As a result, you will need more muscle stability and control of the muscles in your pelvis and back in order to take the stress off the joints.

What about carrying the baby and all the gear?! Without proper muscle support and the ability to recruit from your "core" during these tasks, your spine will take the brunt of the burden, which is what causes that postnatal back pain.

Here are some solutions you can implement today:

1. Set the stroller to the proper height.

If the handlebar height is below elbow height, then you're adding to your troubles and prolonging ill health. At this height, it means that you constantly must lean forward this is, without a doubt, the worst position for maintaining a healthy spine and reducing the occurrence of postnatal back pain. No other position adds more stress to your spine than standing (or walking) while leaning forward. You might be tempted to use the stroller as support, but this will only help for the first few minutes. And if the core muscles are not working like they should, you're likely to suffer long-term problems.

2. Get strong from the inside out.

If, when you lean forward to pick up your own baby, or when you're out for a walk and after only a few minutes you find you need to lean on your baby's stroller for support because your back aches, or you try to go for a jog but can only manage a few minutes until your back hurts, then you've got a problem with your core muscle group that needs fixing fast. If you're suffering from back, groin, or pelvic pain, you need to get the core group of muscles working properly; otherwise, it is very unlikely that you will begin to feel great again.

Learn how to activate your pelvic floor and transverse abdominis with specific exercises like bridges, pelvic tilts, and other "core" activation exercises, not just crunches and planks. This is the one single thing that can help women of ALL AGES, not just with postnatal related back pain.

Note: Sometimes women who have a diastasis recti (abdominal separation) issue that does not heal on its own after about four months postpartum also see an increase in lower postnatal back pain symptoms.

3. Sleep with one pillow.

Any more than one pillow will bend your neck so that the muscles in your back, neck, and shoulders are stretched dangerously more than they are designed to do. You want to keep your neck in a neutral position with your head aligned with your shoulders if possible.

If you do like two pillows, great; the second is best placed between your knees while lying on your side. This will stop your hips from rotating and will help ease back, hip, groin, and pelvic girdle pain.

4. When possible, avoid sitting for longer than 20 minutes.

After nine months of carrying around a baby, you will have weakness in your back. And if you sit for more than 20 minutes, you're stressing your muscles significantly more than they can cope. These muscles are the core group mentioned in principle number one, and if you haven't done anything to retrain them or restore strength, you're adding to your own postnatal back pain problem.

If you are breastfeeding, try placing a pillow or cushion in the small of your back for maximum comfort and support. This is a great temporary fix, but only retraining your core muscle group will allow you to sit safely for more than 20 minutes.

5. Get assessed by a pelvic floor/women's health PT.

Easily, the fastest way to settle back pain is to have it done for you by hand. Most of the time, and on their own, exercises just aren't enough to unlock the problem. If you have joints that have become locked, stiff or stuck during pregnancy, there is only one way for them to become loose — and that's by hand.

The muscles and joints that surround your lower back, pelvic girdle, groin, and hip area will now be very tight and tense. So, manual therapy techniques with massage and joint mobilizations done by a physical therapist will relax them; then these joints would likely be much easier to unlock with the right techniques. When the joints are unlocked, you will feel much freer, looser, more relaxed, and much more like your old active self, especially when followed up by the right types of strengthening exercises.

The techniques that a women's health PT will use prepare the body to work out and exercise, meaning you are going to be much safer, have more movement, feel stronger, and get your energy back fast. And if you can achieve this, you can safely put an end to your worry when leaning over to pick up your own baby. This is even more important if you're 30+ and have had a second child recently, or you're thinking of having another baby sometime soon.

6. Pick up and carry your baby correctly.

One thing you must NOT do is carry your baby on one hip for an extended period of time. You will be adding untold amounts of pressure to your hip, groin, pelvic girdle, and pubic symphysis problems. You need to evenly distribute the weight of your baby as best you can; often, the best way to do this is with a professional carrier or sling. I loved the Baby Ergo (I do not get paid to advertise for them, I just loved the comfort and support of that one).

7. Lift correctly.

Lifting a baby with a weak back is a nightmare for some ladies. Lifting from a low crib is even worse. As baby gains weight, it's even more important to be aware of the way that you lift him or her out of the crib, stroller, or car seat.

The core muscle group absolutely must be strong, but you also need to consider the height of the crib. Is it adjustable? If not, can you position yourself so that when you do lift, your legs aren't completely straight? If they are, your spine is doing all of the work, and long-term back problems await.

So, there you have it, some simple solutions to ease the frustration of your postnatal back pain getting in the way of caring for your family.

For more postnatal back pain tips like this, please visit this special information website: level4pt.com/postnatal-back-pain. *You'll find a free 17-page tips guide waiting for you that shares eight more simple ways to relieve back pain after labor... and feel like yourself again.*

CHAPTER 9

DYSPAREUNIA

Painful Sex

Causes of dyspareunia, also known as painful sex, are commonly misdiagnosed or not diagnosed at all by primary care providers. Often during a gynecological exam, the pain and uncomfortable feeling a woman experiences are just dealt with, or women are told "just relax." This is absurd. An internal exam or sexual intercourse should not be painful. If pain is experienced, then it is highly related to the pelvic floor muscle's function, which is creating increased tension in that area.

Some women have pain during sex for months or even years after childbirth. And some have chronic pain, itching, or burning in their vulva– the tissue surrounding the opening of the vagina.

Client story:

> *Trisha was a 34-year-old mom who called seeking my advice. She had her first baby five months ago after having a C-section. Her abdominals felt weak, but she didn't have any complaints of back pain, and she had good bowel/bladder control. Her biggest complaint was insecurity about having pain the last three times*

she had attempted intercourse with her husband, and she wanted to know how long it would take to feel normal again.

She enjoyed sex before pregnancy, but now it was creating a strain on their intimate relationship. She didn't know what to do. She thought since she didn't have a vaginal delivery, then it didn't make sense for her to still be concerned about her pelvic floor area; it just affected her abdomen, right? After discussing this with her, I let her know an internal assessment would give me a better idea of why she was having so much discomfort. If she couldn't tolerate a pelvic exam, then we would work on strategies to be able to work up to it so she could ease the pain and tension in her pelvic muscles.

With a pelvic floor assessment to check if she had any tender trigger point areas, her muscles appeared strong and able to relax when I gave her some cuing while I had one gloved finger inserted to properly teach her what she was able to control. Then I had her do a couple of breathing exercises to see if I could teach her how to relax her pelvic floor muscles a little more. It was a quick assessment, followed by instructions for what she needed to do to make a difference in relaxing her pelvic muscles over the next few weeks with specific Yoga-based relaxation and stretching exercises and a few PT sessions for some hands-on release of the pelvic floor muscles.

She was happy to have a full description of WHY she was uncomfortable during sex and now had a PLAN to know what she needed to do to improve. Trisha saw me for six visits total; together, we not only cured her painful sex issue, but we fixed some chronic hip pain she had felt over the last ten years!

This is just one example to give you an idea of the power of having the right guidance. Some women are told after complaining of painful intercourse that they should "just relax" or use medication like a vaginal diazepam (really this exists!). But this IS a muscular problem that needs intervention, so you really don't have to struggle with it for the rest of your life and cause a strain on your relationship.

Why did it happen to Trisha? A restricted, painful pelvic floor has a variety of causes. Sometimes, the type of activity you are accustomed to over many years can lead to it. Commonly, ballet dancers, gymnasts, ice skaters, and equestrians are more often the ones with this issue, even prior to pregnancy. This can be attributed to their inherent need to focus on posture and muscle control to perform their sport, sometimes overtraining so much that the internal muscles haven't learned how to release and could be firing "ON" 24/7.

Another cause can be emotional or physical trauma/abuse, which has now created a subconscious holding of the pelvic floor muscles, creating pain like it would with any other muscle that is constantly contracting. Think about a tight muscle in your back; you get tension and pain and feel like you want to stretch it out for relief. Many times, women are subconsciously tense in their pelvic floor, and they are unable to recognize how to relax it. They need to be given verbal and tactile cues to have the awareness to ease it.

I have recently had clients who have undergone a C-section and are now experiencing this type of tension, which could be due to the restriction in the lower abdominal region, area sensitivity, and guarding because of the scar. (Read more in the C-section chapter for additional information.) Vaginal deliveries may lead to this, specifically, because of any tearing in the delivery process, a healing episiotomy scar that is still tender, and so on.

Being instructed on stretching and relaxing techniques that are safe and effective after six weeks postpartum can make a world of difference for this specific issue.

What Can I Do?

1. *Work on relaxation and breathing exercises. Meditation and visualization techniques can also work well. Position yourself on the floor with legs up on a chair and a 90 degree bend in the knee and the hip. Think of inhaling while you fill your belly and your pelvis (down to your vagina) with air. Perform an inhale twice the amount of time the exhale, concentrating on breathing into that pelvis. This is one technique that when resting in this position can get you to relax your hip muscles and pelvic floor while consciously thinking about the breath and where you want it to go. Repeat for 10 minutes at least (as a mom you might just fall asleep too!).*

2. *Next, some Yoga poses are helpful which promote opening of the hips. This includes poses like Happy Baby and Child's Pose with knees apart. Work on the same breathing exercises above, imagining the air moving down into the pelvis on the inhale. Stay relaxed on the exhale. Repeat 10 breaths.*

3. *Finally, with the proper guidance of a pelvic floor PT, the goal is to gently stretch this area and release trigger points that are causing pain. This can be uncomfortable, particularly if you have chronic pain or aren't keen on the idea of internal massage. But a practitioner with whom you feel comfortable will guide you the right way so you don't have to suffer with the problem any longer. This is highly effective for a pelvic floor that does not respond to*

the relaxation poses above and in conjunction with the first two points can be the fastest remedy to help pain with penetration.

Your pelvic floor PT will be gentle and explain every aspect of the treatment before asking your permission to carry on. Any discomfort when your PT presses on tight muscles should not last long. You should have a sense of release or relief afterward when the tightness eases. Each time you are treated with internal/external specific pelvic floor massage or manual therapy treatment, it should become more comfortable. Meditation and relaxation techniques are very helpful for this problem and to help the carryover over improvement after each treatment. For a lot of my clients, it may just take a few treatments to work through this internally; I then follow it up with specific relaxation exercises, Yoga poses (including the two mentioned above) and breath work that address the pelvic floor and allow it to gain long-term relief naturally.

No woman should have to deal with pain during intimacy, and for many women it is not properly diagnosed or even discussed during a medical exam. I hear stories from so many women who were misguided into thinking painful sex was just something they had to deal with or that they just needed to "relax." If your muscles are in a subconscious state of contracting and they haven't been taught how to relax, then it is not possible for it to just happen on its own without professional guidance!

Is this something you have been dealing with?

If you have specific concerns or want to find out more, please visit: level4pt.com/pelvic-pain *(free guide download)*

CHAPTER 10

PELVIC ORGAN PROLAPSE

Breaking the Silence

Do you have a feeling of increased pressure or a feeling of heaviness in the vaginal or rectal area? Maybe you feel like something is out of place and not quite looking the same down there like it used to. Maybe it scared the daylights out of you when you went to the bathroom and you actually saw something poking out. "Wait, was this here before?"

Feelings of frustration and even embarrassment are experienced by many women after not getting the answers they need, and many are often scared of what has changed with their body when experiencing symptoms of prolapse. This is what I hear from my clients who ask if this is something that is normal after labor and delivery.

Some women experience symptoms within weeks of delivering, while others reach their 50s and 60s and never even knew this was a risk after years of lifting, pushing, pulling, and doing activities with a weak core and pelvic floor. Some were considering surgery because their doctors said that was the solution.

"This can happen to me?"

When pregnancy and childbirth weaken or stretch the pelvic floor muscles and the surrounding tissue, one or more of the organs they support – the uterus, bladder, and bowel – can bulge into the vagina. This is called prolapse. Some women experience a prolapse after childbirth when the structures that support the pelvic organs are weakened. Usually, both a muscular portion and ligaments that support the organs can no longer perform properly. A common reason for this to happen is that the muscles are damaged during the act of childbirth and also as a result of the pressure that pregnancy puts on a woman's body. Despite popular belief, it is an inaccurate assumption that uterine prolapse exclusively affects only older women.

Symptoms of prolapse:

- *the feeling of pressure or heaviness in the vagina or rectal area*
- *a distinct bulge (or lump) inside or protruding from the vagina*
- *feeling of incomplete emptying*
- *poor or prolonged urinary stream*
- *position changes needed to start or complete emptying*
- *pain during sexual intercourse*

The different types of prolapse:

- *Cystocele–Bladder*
- *Urethrocele–Urethra*
- *Urethrocystocele–Urethra and Bladder*
- *Uterine Prolapse–Uterine*
- *Rectocele–Rectum*
- *Enterocele–Small intestine*

- *Vaginal vault prolapse–Vagina*
- *Rectal prolapse–Rectrum*

There are four stages to a prolapse, which is important for women to understand and indicates the extent to which the uterus has descended. It is possible that the bladder and bowel, as part of a group of pelvic organs, may also drop as a result of the prolapse.

The FOUR STAGES ARE (and in this case we are using uterine prolapse as the example):

Stage 1: The uterus has descended into the upper part of the vagina.

Stage 2: The uterus is almost at the vaginal opening.

Stage 3: The uterus is protruding from the vagina.

Stage 4: The uterus has descended to the point where it is entirely outside the vagina.

*Prolapse is common in older women, but it can affect younger women who've experienced a long and complicated labor, had a large baby, or had multiple babies. **Recently, it has been more common in women who return to high intensity exercise like running and heavy weight lifting too soon without strengthening the internal muscles and fully recovering after labor and delivery.***

Some moms worry that they have prolapse when, in fact, they have a weak pelvic floor and slackness in the surrounding muscles. When you are unable to support your muscles, you often get a "dragging" feeling in your vagina. This will go away or reduce as your pelvic floor regains strength. With pelvic floor rehabilitation, you can often get your pelvic floor working again to minimize the symptoms of the prolapse. Surgery is NOT always necessary, and working with a good pelvic floor PT can significantly minimize symptoms and allow you to have an active life that you once feared wasn't going to be possible.

Pelvic floor muscles can be made weaker by:

- *not keeping them active;*
- *being pregnant and having babies;*
- *constipation;*
- *being overweight;*
- *heavy lifting;*
- *coughing that goes on for a long time (such as smoker's cough, bronchitis or asthma);*
- *and menopause (hormonal changes).*

Client story with prolapse:

> *Veronica is a 55-year-old female who had been feeling increased pressure and heaviness in her pelvic area. She wanted to stay active, but was concerned symptoms would worsen and would continue to affect her as she reached her 60s and 70s. She was even experiencing cramping-like feeling in her lower abdominal region, and it made her anxious because she didn't know the cause.*
>
> *After multiple visits, her doctor told her that she had a prolapse and gave her the option of using a device called a pessary that would help hold it in place. This was very uncomfortable and she decided to do some research on her own, which led her to read about pelvic floor PT. She had been working on Kegel exercises with little change in her symptoms over the past year. Her kids were now in*

their 20s, and she asked me, "Isn't it too late for me? I was told surgery could fix this."

An assessment revealed she had a very weak pelvic floor, unable to activate her muscles without compensating with her glutes and inner thighs. Additionally, every Kegel contraction she performed caused her to push out her abdominals and hold her breath. We worked on correcting this for once a week for the next six weeks, giving her cuing and exercises to work on in between sessions, and in a short amount of time she was so relieved to have a renewed sense of confidence about her body. The cramping symptoms went away, her back felt even stronger, and she experienced no more heaviness/pressure in the pelvic area. She said it really was amazing, and she was sorry she had waited so long to come get my help!

Why is Veronica's story so common? I hear this time and time again, women who go about life thinking this is just the way it has to be, not taking action to help themselves. The reason I included Veronica's story was to show you that it can happen to women of all ages, and conservative interventions can make a world of difference.

For many women prolapse can be an effect of a dysfunctional pelvic floor. I could tell you the answer is "go do more Kegel exercises", but that is not often the case. To give you a simple solution for helping a prolapse and to get the BEST outcome, you need to see a good pelvic floor PT. This way you can find out if your muscles are really just weak, shortened or tight and have trouble protecting the organs, OR if there is a poor connection between knowing how to actually get the muscles to work when you need them!

I can't emphasize enough the importance of consulting with a pelvic floor PT if you have any of these symptoms above or if you have been told you have a prolapse. I would be doing a dis-service if I told you there is a "take home" solution, but it is very individualized. Very commonly, an OB or gynecologist will not normally assess for a prolapse unless you ask, and, even more often, a pelvic floor PT will not be a recommendation from an OB/GYN. But, now that you are reading this book, you know that pelvic floor PTs specialize in treating prolapse!

CHAPTER 11

C-SECTION

Belly Births and Scar Care

So, you had a C-section (or, as we love to call it, a "Belly Birth"). Information for what to do in the first six weeks is easily accessible–how to be careful lifting and taking it easy, resting, etc. But what do you do for exercise now that your OB/GYN cleared you at that six- to eight-week mark and said your scar is "healed"? Talking about C-section recovery is almost non-existent; resources are NOT given to moms to address incision care, scar massage, exercise progression, etc. Most women are only told not to lift anything, drive, or exercise for six weeks post C-section (or post hysterectomy), even though they had major abdominal and pelvic surgery. That's it? That is all the information they get?

C-sections are common, accounting for an estimated 31.9 percent of all deliveries in the United States. It is important to know that not all women will heal at the same rate and be ready for the same activity after surgery, even though most of the information out there relates to healing by six to eight weeks post C-section. Setting reasonable expectations and having a supportive medical team can make the recovery from a C-section easier.

Some studies, for example, have found that 60 percent of women have some pain in the incision 24 weeks after delivery.[10]

Here is a story about a recent client of mine who was having this specific issue:

Jessica's story:

> *Jessica is a 32-year-old mom who knew she would have a C-section at 39.5 weeks because she was told her baby was breech. This was her first baby, and when she was told she needed a C-section, she didn't quite know what to expect. Jessica and the baby both did well during the delivery process and followed the nurses' and doctor's instructions in the hospital and early weeks at home with the initial instructions. What she didn't expect is that simple tasks would be challenging, like taking a shower on her own, caring for the baby, etc., so she asked for help at home, plus she hired a postpartum doula (great thinking!).*

> *At the six-week checkup with her OB, Jessica was told her incision was healed, she did great, and to go back gradually to her activities. What she didn't expect was that the pain in her abdominal area would still continue post C-section after six weeks.*

For most people following a knee or shoulder surgery, the surgeon would commonly recommend PT as a follow up to progressively work on moving again and strengthening. This is just not the case for abdominal surgery— and that's just crazy! I want YOU to be confident in your ability to

---

[10] National Collaborating Centre for Womens and Childrens Health. *Caesarean Section (NICE Clinical Guideline 132). Royal College of Obstetrics and Gynaecology, 2011.*

facilitate your recovery, and I want to help you return to exercise safely and strongly.

Your OB clears you post C-section and you are healed in six weeks?

NOT SO FAST!

As you can tell from this description, a C-section is not the gentlest of procedures on the body and organs, so adequate rest and recovery are essential. YOU need to be patient with the process and not push through it. It's possible that you had a C-section, and weeks, months, or even years later you're still dealing with pain around or beneath the incision site, a weakness in your abdominal region, and fear about touching your scar.

Physiological healing time for any body part is about six to eight weeks; that means your cervix and uterus most likely have recovered to their former pre-pregnancy position and size. For some women, the scar is sensitive to touch, or it feels numb. A pelvic floor PT can teach you specific techniques to promote healing, such as moving the scar up and down perpendicularly with your index fingers, moving in a circular motion gently along the scar, and also at a 45-degree angle to work on the scar tissue; this will help to prevent the formation of adhesions and is so important after the incision is closed. Abdominal and pelvic adhesions can be side effects of a C-section.

Often times, the abdominal area can feel numb or disconnected even weeks to months after a C-section. Learning how to sensitize the area again with massage techniques plus how to engage the abdominal and pelvic floor muscles can make a world of difference to feeling like you are getting your strength back again.

Abdominal adhesions are a common complication of surgery, occurring in a majority of people who undergo abdominal or pelvic surgery. Most adhesions are painless and do not cause complications. However, adhesions can contribute to the development of chronic pelvic pain.

- *Adhesions typically begin to form within the first few days after surgery, but they may not produce symptoms for months or even years. As scar tissue begins to restrict motion of the small intestines, it may even cause problems in the digestive system.*

- *In extreme cases, adhesions may form fibrous bands around an entire segment of the intestine; this constricts blood flow and can lead to tissue death. A non-invasive way to treat these adhesions includes manual soft tissue bodywork by a PT to decrease the symptoms.*

Pelvic adhesions may involve any organ within the pelvis, such as the uterus, ovaries, Fallopian tubes, or bladder, and usually occur after a C-section or hysterectomy, sometimes causing painful sex.

"I didn't have a vaginal birth, so my pelvic floor is fine." *The fact is that 43 percent of those who deliver via cesarean section have a pelvic floor dysfunction (compared to 58 percent of women who deliver vaginally). Many patients I have seen after a C-section had pelvic floor symptoms relating to either painful sex or incontinence, and here are some reasons for this:*

- *The downward pressure of the baby can stretch the pelvic floor muscles and their connective tissues, leaving them more lax than normal.*

- *The expanding uterus puts pressure on other pelvic organs, including the bladder and the rectum, and can disrupt their normal function.*

- *C-section scars can sometimes create strange nerve-like symptoms, leading to side effects like urethral burning, the feeling of needing to pee all the time, and pain in the clitoris and labia.*

- *A C-section is often necessary in the case of a multiple baby birth (twins, triplets, etc.), which has increased the pressure with heavier weight on the pelvic floor during pregnancy.*

- *The alignment changes that happen during pregnancy and postpartum, like having your pelvis shifted forward or tucked under, can affect the tone of your pelvic floor muscles, leaving them tight and short.*

If you have tight muscles, you may continue to feel pain, even after your wound has healed. If you have an overactive pelvic floor, or your muscles are used to working in overdrive, helpful treatment from a pelvic floor PT can provide trigger point massage or trigger point release internally to relax the muscles and ease internal pelvic pain.

(See Chapter 9 for causes of and solutions to painful sex.)

Trigger point release is similar to any other massage, with the main difference being that the pelvic floor can be massaged internally. Trigger point release identifies sensitive points, and it helps your muscles to relax and move naturally after time. A pelvic floor PT will use her gloved index finger to massage the tender areas in order to release the muscle and create more tissue inside your vagina.

If you think of any other tender muscles in the body, offering pressure and massage to the area is a treatment to relieve the discomfort and create more blood flow and circulation to the area, thereby allowing the muscle to return to its natural state. This also will affect the ability of the muscle to contract more efficiently.

Although the doctor might clear you for post C-section exercise six to eight weeks after surgery, be certain this means light, gentle exercise. Exercises that may be beneficial at this time include breathing, walking, core restoration, and bodyweight exercises. Exercises that are not beneficial at this time are, for example, running, jumping, heavy weight training, crunches, leg raises, and other traditional abdominal exercises. But what should you start first?

It's important to understand why jumping back into high intensity exercises at six to eight weeks is not recommended and what you can do to BUILD up to it!

Here is the process:

During a C-section, the doctor makes an incision into the skin, through the fat cells and connective tissue, and into the abdominal cavity. The abdominal muscles are spread apart, and the bladder is moved down and out of the way in order to reach the uterus. An incision is made into the uterus, and the baby is guided out. The placenta is taken out shortly after. The uterus is stitched up, the bladder put back in place, and the skin is sutured. Due to the many layers of sutures, scar tissue will form.

Initial recommendations for the first six weeks post C-section:

1. Get plenty of rest.

Rest is vital for recovery from any surgery, yet for many new parents, rest is nearly impossible with a newborn in the home. Newborns keep irregular hours and may sleep for only one or two hours at a time.

People should always try to sleep when the baby sleeps or take a nap while a loved one helps.

It is easy to feel overwhelmed by chores or to want to entertain visitors, but giving up sleep to put away dishes or keep the house clean can be damaging to someone's health. It is more sensible to try to sleep as much as possible.

2. Ask for help.

Newborns are demanding. Caring for a baby after major surgery can be exhausting, and it is not possible for all new parents to manage this alone. Ask for help from a partner, a neighbor, family, or a trusted friend.

People may benefit from lining up a meal train or a schedule of visitors who can watch the baby while you rest or take a shower.

3. Process your emotions.

Giving birth can be an emotional time. Women who experience emergency deliveries or traumatic births, as well as those who have cesarean deliveries they hoped to avoid, may have to process difficult emotions about the birth. These new feelings can make the transition to parenthood more difficult than it is for others, and they can trigger new feelings.

Talk to a partner, friend, or therapist. Getting early support may help reduce the risk of postpartum depression and can help women experiencing postpartum depression get quicker treatment. Movement and walking, while getting outside, can be a huge help for your emotional wellbeing (see #4).

4. Take regular walks.

Lifting and intense aerobic exercise are out for the first few weeks of recovery. As an alternative, walking can help with staying fit and maintaining good mental health.

Taking a walk also reduces the risk of blood clots and other heart or blood vessel issues. Some new parents like walking with other new parents as part of a group, or they prefer meeting up with a neighbor to push their babies in their strollers.

5. Manage pain.

There is no need to be in pain while struggling with all the other demands of new parenting; people must take the pain relievers prescribed by their doctor. If they do not work or if the pain gets worse, they should contact a health care provider for advice.

6. Watch for signs of infection.

Some doctors will ask new parents to take their own temperature every 24 hours to monitor for signs of infection. You can consult with your doctor or midwife to ask if this is a good strategy.

Also, new mothers must be mindful of other signs of infection, such as swelling, intense pain, red streaks coming from the incision, or chills. Contact a doctor or go to the emergency room if these symptoms appear.

7. Fight constipation.

The combination of hormonal shifts, weaker stomach muscles, and spending large quantities of time lying down can lead to constipation, so you want to move. Severe constipation can be painful, and straining can injure the C-section incision.

Drink plenty of water, and ask a doctor about taking a stool softener. Eating plenty of fiber-rich foods, such as fruit and vegetables, can help to prevent constipation.

8. Get support for breastfeeding.

Having a C-section may be linked to a higher risk of breastfeeding difficulties. A lactation consultant can help new parents successfully breastfeed, even when they face obstacles, such as separation from the baby after birth. If breastfeeding is not going well, mothers should ask for help. If you are local to San Diego, I have a referral list for you.

If you are in pain, sitting in a comfortable, supportive chair and using a breastfeeding cushion, or nursing in a laid-back, reclining position can make breastfeeding easier.

9. Seek help for long-term issues.

Here's where all women should seek out help from a specialized pelvic floor PT post C-section. It is very common to experience muscle weakness, incontinence, or depression, and mothers should not feel ashamed if they have these symptoms; nor is there any need to suffer in silence. Referring you to a practitioner who can help guide you through this process is hugely important.

You can learn many strategies for recovering from childbirth from visiting a pelvic floor PT; hearing about these strategies after your OB/GYN checkup should be a normal occurrence, but they are not always suggested. You can receive guidance on the appropriate transitioning to exercise, reducing bowel and pelvic floor over activity, and improving scar tissue mobility to prevent further pain/difficulty with abdominal healing.

Move on to the conclusion to learn what action steps you can take right now!

CHAPTER 12

EXERCISE

How Busy Moms Can Find Time

*Sticking with an exercise routine can be a struggle for anyone, but squeezing in workouts can feel darn near impossible for moms. After all, how are you supposed to find time to work out when you can't even go to the bathroom undisturbed? And that's not even considering all of the postpartum issues some moms have to deal with by themselves. **But they don't have to deal with this alone, and that's where I come in as a women's health and pelvic floor PT. We are the doctors that most women are never told to see, even though we are perhaps the ones they need to see most. At least that's the case in the United States.***

Between caring for kids, workplace demands, household chores, doctor appointments, school, and all the rest, precious little time remains for moms to sweat. So, I wanted to share with you some of my best tips for making exercise a reality and a priority. (It's possible. I swear!) And if your child is under the age of two, my advice is SLEEP FIRST! ...then consider these!

1. Put first things first.

Work out before the day gets away from you. If I waited until after work, I'd never get my workout in; too many activities and commitments compete for my attention. No one will schedule a meeting at 5:30 a.m.; that's your time to sweat. Another reason to sweat early is that you're finished before the kids wake up!

2. Block it out.

If you have an appointment on your calendar, chances are you show up; that same tactic will help you find time for your sweat sessions. If you set aside specific times in your planner, they feel more like an appointment you have to keep. Each Sunday, manage your family's calendar. I block out "Dawn goes to yoga" on Thursday nights, so my husband knows it's his night to pick up our daughters and prepare dinner. I do the same for him. Schedule it as part of your day and make it non-negotiable.

3. Have a plan for how you'll sweat.

Once you've penciled in your workout, don't forget to think about what you'll actually do once you get to the gym. It's one thing to find the motivation to work out; it's another thing to find the motivation to figure out what to do for a workout. If you know beforehand exactly what you plan to do, you make it happen.

4. Don't worry about your outfit.

Printed capris or plain black? Tank top or t-shirt? Don't waste your little free time debating wardrobe choices. To make it to your early morning workout, lay out your clothes the night before. Heck, sleep in your workout clothes if that helps! Eliminating that one step of figuring out what to wear makes getting up at 5 a.m. easier.

5. Include your kids.

It's hard to find dedicated "alone time" as a parent—but do you really need it? I struggled with finding time to work out alone without the kids. I quickly learned that wasn't always possible. I've embraced working out with my girls, and they see that I am a strong woman who enjoys working out. You should ditch the "either-or" attitude. Children instinctively love to move. Resistance bands are great for playing "hop over," and BOSU balls make fun mini trampolines. As your children grow older, workouts can be bonding time. I've always made a point of introducing my daughters to fitness. Now my oldest daughter runs with me a few times a week, and we've already run our first 5k and Thanksgiving "turkey trot" together.

6. Make the jungle gym your bootcamp.

Who says that you're too old to play outside? I remember taking our daughters to the playground, and I played right along with them. A game of tag or freeze tag anyone? I'll do triceps dips off a bench, incline push-ups, step ups on a bench, and try to do a pull-up on the monkey bars. Those little bursts of activity do add up quickly!

7. Run with them.

When your children's increasingly early wake-up times threaten to ruin your early morning jog, run with them. I remember placing them in the jogging stroller and taking them with me. I'd sing and chat during our run together. Instead of spoiling my run, it just made it a little bit sweeter. It may require a bit more planning since the kids have to be dressed and you have to pack snacks, books and drinks, but it's a great way to spend time with them while exercising.

8. Take to the streets.

Being a soccer mom in a minivan is cliché—so ditch the ride. Since we live in San Diego and weather permits nearly year-round, we make our commute an active one. Attempt to walk your kids to school, or bike to work. We live about a half-mile from our daughters' elementary school, so if the weather is nice we can base exercise on trips to and from school.

9. Audit your schedule.

Regular exercisers don't find time, they "take" time. Most of us have unused chunks of time in our day—30-minutes spent on Facebook or Instagram, 10-minute intervals spent checking email or cleaning. Pay attention to how you're spending your time, and figure out from which activities you could "take" time. If possible, lump all those chunks together and use them for a workout. If not, spread your activity throughout the day.

10. Music class is for them; gym class is for you.

Between soccer practice, ballet, or music lessons, kids are sometimes as busy as their parents these days. Use the time that your kids are in classes wisely. Your kids are getting their fitness in, why shouldn't you? While my daughters are at soccer practice, I squeeze in time on the track. My kids decompress from their school day, get some exercise, and connect with their friends on the soccer field—and I get to do the same on the track. Naptime is another prime time to squeeze in a workout. As soon as your kids go down for a nap, leave them with Dad and go out for a run or to the gym. Usually, you'll be back by the time they wake up and everyone is refreshed.

11. Don't beat yourself up.

Let's face it, life happens in the form of sick days, tantrums, and gigantic messes that won't clean themselves. Some days I only have time for a few *miles instead of the planned five or six miles on my training plan. Learn to accept the time you do have, and make the most of it. The next day, I might run the miles faster than planned or run a few more miles to make up for it. If you do miss a day, don't stress. Don't compare yourself to other moms. Do your best for you.*

12. Make any space a home gym.

While not making it to the gym or a class is a convenient excuse, the truth is, you don't need special fitness equipment or a gym membership to work out. If you're truly stuck at home, use what you have at your disposal. Sometimes it's nothing more than a chair, but you'd be surprised at the range of exercises you can do with a chair!

13. Make it worth it.

At the end of the day, spending more time with your family is always a priority. Working full-time, traveling, running a business, and everything else means less time with my children. One of the mantras I've adopted is: "Make it worth it." If you're going to choose to run or go to the gym rather than spend time with your children, you better make sure you're pushing yourself the entire time.

So, there you have 13 of my best tips on how busy moms can find time to exercise. The excuses are many, but only if you let yourself make them. I understand fitting fitness into a busy schedule is hard, and exercise is often the first thing to get scratched from the calendar. But, with a little forethought and planning, it's doable. Make your well-being a priority.

Just don't allow yourself to think of your health as a secondary priority. When you are happy and healthy, everyone else has a better shot of following suit.

CONCLUSION

Moms, Let's Take Action!

What you can do NOW to improve your pelvic health

If you are experiencing ANY of the issues that you read about so far in this book, I urge you to take these simple steps!

1. Look up "Pelvic Floor Physical Therapist" in your area (this is one good way to use Google). Then ask if you can speak to a specialist first, or do a free consultation to get more information. In most cases in the USA no referral from a medical doctor is required. If no one will give you information or allow you to speak to a specialist first, then it is probably not the best facility for you to visit. My office is in northern San Diego, but we are happy to find a resource closer to you if you live outside of the area. Just know that sometimes your OB or GYN will not always recommend this option, and it's likely because they might not truly understand how we can help you. Seeking out a pelvic floor PT is the #1 most important way to get individualized and specialized care!

2. Start working on your pelvic floor muscles and testing your ability to do the following simple exercises (NOTE: if you are experiencing painful sex as described in Chapter 7, these may not be the right exercises for you, yet. Get checked first):

Elevator breathing and control of pelvic floor: Take it up a level by starting this exercise rather than by starting with a general Kegel. Imagine your pelvic floor muscles as part of a three-story building with an elevator.

   a. *Imagine the doors of the elevator closing as you squeeze your pelvic floor muscles, then lift from the vaginal area like an elevator moving up to level one of the building (about 30 percent of your pressure).*

   b. *Hold there.*

   c. *Then imagine the elevator lifting to the second floor by lifting the pelvic floor muscles another 30 percent (or about 60 percent of your total pressure).*

   d. *Hold there for a couple of seconds.*

   e. *Then imagine lifting up the pelvic floor muscles via elevator to the third floor at 100 percent of your full strength, and see if you can hold another two to three seconds.*

   f. *Now relax the pelvic floor down to the ground floor where you started with full relaxation.*

   g. *Repeat five times.*

3. *Return to Chapter 4 and go through the* **timeline for restorative exercises** *(especially my top five postnatal exercises). If you do this for three weeks and are not pleased with how you feel, or if you are doing something similar already but your symptoms have not resolved, please take my advice in #1 above to find a pelvic floor PT.*

If you are dealing with the internal struggle of thinking your post-pregnancy life will always be like this, then I hope you were able to get some clarity by reading this book. Maybe you realized you are not alone and that a resource exists to help guide you in the right direction. If you are a woman who fears surgery, who worries that she will continue to feel discomfort for the next two years, who doesn't feel right about taking medications to manage an issue, or who just wants to feel stronger and more confident about her body, then this book was written for you!

I would love to explain many more details in this book, but I did touch on the main topics that elicit the most questions and that would make the most impact on my readers. My biggest accomplishment with this book was providing valuable information for women of all ages; it offers guidance on topics that have scant resources, and it gives direction to fix common physical issues suffered by so many active women.

The reason I took this career path was to help guide women who were falling through gaps in the healthcare system. Before reading this book, you might not have realized what a pelvic floor PT even was or why you would need to visit one. My biggest hope is that you find the information that may lead you down the path to improved health and wellness.

The next most important step to get your problem resolved is to find a pelvic floor PT who will give you the time to really be heard and clearly educate you on your particular issue, will be able to address the issue with a full-body approach, and will get to the root of your problem so you can reach your goals. Visit our website for more information about how to find the best PT for you: level4pt.com/about/

I know how busy life is as a mom since I am doing it myself, but I also know that you might be dealing with a physical issue that has put unwanted stress on your marriage, has affected the way you feel about yourself, and impacted your ability to stay as active as you would like to be. Just know that even if it has been years since you delivered your baby, you will make such a huge gain by taking some of the action steps in this book right now. I see women in their 40s, 50s, and beyond who wish they had known about the pelvic floor and the importance it plays in bladder/bowel function, sexual health, fitness and life performance, and reducing prolapse symptoms.

The tips in this book have been used on me and on thousands of clients I have worked with in person and virtually. So, go back to the chapter that kept your attention the most and read it again; then take action, and use the tips given. If you need guidance or have questions, please visit level4pt.com/womens-health for a variety of helpful resources.

Thanks for reading!

GET YOUR FREE WOMEN'S HEALTH GIFT
FROM THE LEVEL4 SPECIALISTS, NOW...

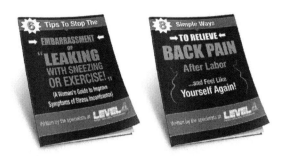

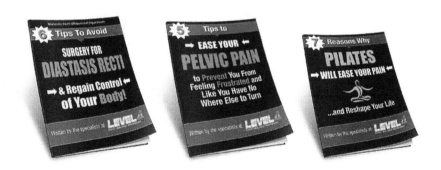

Go to **level4pt.com/womens-health-gifts/**
Claim your $500 worth of health tips which have helped 1000s of women
feel more confident and strong postpartum...so they can continue living the
active lifestyle they want...and deserve, absolutely FREE!
Claim your copies now!

level4pt.com/womens-health-gifts/

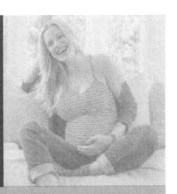
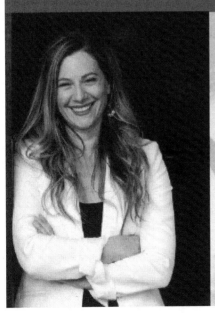
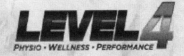

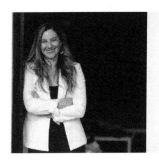

Helping Active Women
Regain Confidence In Their Body, Stay Active
and Strong .. So They Can Feel Like
Themselves Again.
(No Matter What Age!)

Online Coaching From Dr. Dawn at LEVEL4 - Leading Expert In Women's Health & Fitness - And Guiding You Safely Back To Weightlifting, Running and HIIT Style Workouts Post-Pregnancy

This Program Is For You If...

- *You are a mom who plans on Returning to High Intensity Exercise such as running, weight lifting, jumping activities, and core exercises (no matter how fit you think you were leading up to pregnancy and during!)*
- *You are scared to do the exercises (especially the abdominal ones) you used to do and not sure how to start your fitness program (even though your doctor said you are cleared for exercise)*
- *You love to follow a fitness program where someone is telling you what to do week by week!*
- *You want guidance from a specialist who can help you PREVENT "leaking" with jumping, sneezing, and running, help HEAL and RESTORE your CORE AND PELVIC FLOOR so you CAN feel confident about returning to exercise, and help PREVENT pelvic organ prolapse (which is more common than you think with a dysfunctional pelvic floor!)*
- *Learn more than just KEGELS or PLANKS for restoring your pelvic floor and abdominals*

SIGN UP FOR A FREE VIRTUAL CALL:
level4pt.com/beyond-9-months/

NOTES

1. Declercq E. R. et al. *Listening to mothers: Report of the first national U.S. survey of women's childbearing experiences.* New York: Maternity Center Association, 2002.

2. Thompson, Jane F., et al. "Prevalence and Persistence of Health Problems After Childbirth: Associations with Parity and Method of Birth." *Birth,* vol. 29, no. 2, 16 May 2002, pp. 83–94., doi:10.1046/j.1523-536x.2002.00167.x.

3. Cheng, Ching-Yu, et al. "Postpartum Maternal Health Care in the United States: A Critical Review." *Journal of Perinatal Education,* vol. 15, no. 3, 2006, pp. 34–42., doi:10.1624/105812406x119002.

4. Vries, Raymond De, et al. *Birth by Design: Pregnancy, Maternity Care, and Midwifery in North America and Europe.* Routledge, 2001.

5. Tarkka, Marja-Terttu, et al. "Social Support Provided by Public Health Nurses and the Coping of First-Time Mothers with Child Care." *Public Health Nursing,* vol. 16, no. 2, 1999, pp. 114–119., doi:10.1046/j.1525-1446.1999.00114.x.

6. Harvard Health Publishing. "In the Journals: Pelvic Floor Muscle Training Can Help Reverse Pelvic Organ Prolapse." *Harvard Health,* Jan. 2011, https://www.health.harvard.edu/womens-health/pelvic-floor-muscle-training-can-help-reverse-pelvic-organ-prolapse.

7. Nakamura, Aurélie, et al. "Physical Activity during Pregnancy and Postpartum Depression: Systematic Review and Meta-Analysis."

Journal of Affective Disorders, vol. 246, 2019, pp. 29–41., doi:10.1016/j.jad.2018.12.009.

8. Nygaard, Ingrid, et al. "Exercise and Incontinence." *Obstetrics and Gynecology,* vol. 75, no. 5, May 1990, pp. 848–851, journals.lww.com/greenjournal/Abstract/1990/05000/Exercise_and_In continence.26.aspx#pdf-link.

9. Cavkaytar, S., et al. "Effect of Home-Based Kegel Exercises on Quality of Life in Women with Stress and Mixed Urinary Incontinence." *Journal of Obstetrics and Gynaecology,* vol. 35, no. 4, 2014, pp. 407–407, doi:10.3109/01443615.2014.960831.